AF806238

57-
WPS
20

Community Quality-of-Life and Well-Being

Series Editor

Rhonda Phillips, Purdue University, West Lafayette, IN, USA

The Community Quality of Life and Well-being book series is a collection of volumes related to community level research, providing community planners and quality of life researchers involved in community and regional well-being innovative research and application. Formerly entitled, Community Quality of Life Indicators: Best Practices, the series reflects a broad scope of well-being. Next to best practices of community quality-of-life indicators projects the series welcomes a variety of research and practice topics as related to overall community well-being and quality of life dimensions, whether relating to policy, application, research, and/or practice. Research on issues such as societal happiness, quality of life domains in the policy construct, measuring and gauging progress, dimensions of planning and community development, and related topics are anticipated. This series is published by Springer in partnership with the International Society for Quality-of-Life Studies, a global society with the purpose of promoting and encouraging research and collaboration in quality of life and well-being theory and applications.

More information about this series at http://www.springer.com/series/13761

Youngwha Kee · Seung Jong Lee ·
Rhonda Phillips
Editors

Perspectives on Community Well-Being

Springer

Mängelexemplar

Editors
Youngwha Kee
Soongsil University
Seoul, Korea (Republic of)

Seung Jong Lee
Seoul National University
Seoul, Korea (Republic of)

Rhonda Phillips
Honors College
Purdue University
West Lafayette, IN, USA

ISSN 2520-1093 ISSN 2520-1107 (electronic)
Community Quality-of-Life and Well-Being
ISBN 978-3-030-15114-0 ISBN 978-3-030-15115-7 (eBook)
https://doi.org/10.1007/978-3-030-15115-7

Library of Congress Control Number: 2019935533

© Springer Nature Switzerland AG 2019
This work is subject to copyright. All rights are reserved by the Publisher, whether the whole or part of the material is concerned, specifically the rights of translation, reprinting, reuse of illustrations, recitation, broadcasting, reproduction on microfilms or in any other physical way, and transmission or information storage and retrieval, electronic adaptation, computer software, or by similar or dissimilar methodology now known or hereafter developed.
The use of general descriptive names, registered names, trademarks, service marks, etc. in this publication does not imply, even in the absence of a specific statement, that such names are exempt from the relevant protective laws and regulations and therefore free for general use.
The publisher, the authors and the editors are safe to assume that the advice and information in this book are believed to be true and accurate at the date of publication. Neither the publisher nor the authors or the editors give a warranty, expressed or implied, with respect to the material contained herein or for any errors or omissions that may have been made. The publisher remains neutral with regard to jurisdictional claims in published maps and institutional affiliations.

This Springer imprint is published by the registered company Springer Nature Switzerland AG
The registered company address is: Gewerbestrasse 11, 6330 Cham, Switzerland

Preface

This volume provides a variety of perspectives on community well-being, from different disciplines, cultures, and frameworks. It encompasses several chapters from a conference of the International Society for Quality-of-Life Studies www.isqols.org, and convenings of the Community Well-Being Research Center, housed in Korea, www.communitywellbeing.org. Researchers from around the globe have contributed to this volume, which serves as the fourth book contribution by the editors to the topic of community well-being.[1] This is an area of growing interest that encapsulates dimensions of well-being and quality of life across a range of domains and considerations—whether from the perspective of governance, resident participation, community development, learning, or a host of myriad other influences on community well-being. Our focus is predominately on communities of place, and collectives (or what some may call communities of interest) within those places; it is also about the governing of these places, as reflected in policy and programming by local governments to explore or foster enhanced well-being.

This will be the fourth volume we have completed on community well-being, an area of interest and research that is rapidly evolving. The need for research on this topic is very high, and interest continues to accelerate. This proposed volume brings together multiple diverse perspectives on quality of life and community well-being. The purpose of this volume is to present this collection across disciplines, ideas, and perspectives to foster more interest and research in community well-being. *Perspectives on Community Well-Being* provides various insights on quality of life and well-being from a place-based perspective. Topics include surveying at the community level, child-friendly communities, collective impact, grieving, and

[1]The other three books by the editors are: Youngwha Kee, Seung Jong Lee, and Rhonda Phillips. (eds.) (2016). *Social Factors and Community Well-Being*. Dordrecht, The Netherlands: Springer. www.springer.com/us/book/9783319299402; Seung Jong Lee, Yunji Kim and Rhonda Phillips. (eds.) (2015). *Community Well-Being and Community Development*, Dordrecht, The Netherlands: Springer. www.springer.com/social+sciences/wellbeing+%26+quality-of-life/book/978-3-319-12420-9; and Youngwha Kee, Yunji Kim and Rhonda Phillips. (eds.) (2015). *Learning and Community Applications for Promoting Well-Being*, Dordrecht, The Netherlands: Springer. www.springer.com/social+sciences/wellbeing+%26+quality-of-life/book/978-3-319-12438-4.

happiness. This edited volume brings together perspectives from around the globe and provides both conceptual and applied explorations. Those working in the areas of public policy, community development, community and social psychology, as well as planning and development will find this volume particularly useful for the array of perspectives, research, and analytical approaches presented.

Certainly, many aspects of an area can influence community well-being, which can include "comprehensive and integrated concepts developed by synthesizing research constructs related to residents' perceptions of the community, resident's needs fulfillment, observable community conditions, and the social and cultural context of the community" (Sung and Phillips 2016: 2). Along this same line of thinking, Haworth and Hart (2007: 95) explain community well-being as "focused on understanding the contribution of a community in maintaining itself and fulfilling the various needs of local residents." This communal aspect is especially important and considered to be a contributing aspect of social organizations and relationships; it can be considered as "something that we do together, not something that we each possess" (p. 128).

Community well-being is a complex, interconnected concept, and it is gaining increasing interest as a framework that can help explain "quality of life and happiness in a communal context, than that on an individual level" (Kee and Nam 2016: 39). It is sometimes described as an umbrella concept, branching out over several related aspects of collective living—community development, happiness, quality of life, sustainability, and other allied constructs or approaches influencing well-being—both abstract and multidimensional (Lee, Kim & Phillips 2015: 2). In this way, community well-being can be considered as "embedded with multidimensional values including the economic, social, and environmental aspects that impact people" (Phillips and Wong 2017: xxix). It is similar in concept to ideas around sustainability that encompass major dimensions or domains of life—environment, economic, and equity (social/cultural and related). Given these multiple ways to influence well-being, whether via the physical environment, economic and social conditions, health, and type of governance structure, there exists a rich array of approaches, cases, and frameworks for community well-being.

This volume provides a collection of such a rich array, with views and insight offered across a panoply of perspectives and applications. Chapter 1 begins with an exploration of how to measure and gauge happiness by Kai Ludwigs, Lena Henning, and Lidia Arends. Happiness is a vital aspect of community well-being and they begin by explaining that happiness research remains a young discipline with definitions unclear across various disciplines, with many different measurement techniques having been developed. They present a definition by the World Database of Happiness, and then present a comprehensive review of measurements for evaluating happiness. This is an extensive chapter that provides much needed delineation of concepts of happiness, in the context of community-level well-being. They conclude with an applied guideline for researchers to consider when measuring happiness.

Chapter 2, "An Indigenous Perspective on Quality of Life", by Pat Lauderdale provides a view of the interrelatedness of nature. Written from the perspective of indigenous peoples, it considers these relationships in the context of striving for improved well-being and quality of life. Traditional indigenous knowledge is held as holding much "potential for long-lasting approaches to current environment problems and provide us with ideas on how to improve our questions and, therefore, improve our potential for more equitable, less oppressive structures from which to approach the numerous problems." There is a powerful lesson here—that we focus on learning from the deep interconnection we share with nature, respecting it while learning from it as is tradition by indigenous peoples.

Our third selection is "A Participatory Process: Creating Child Friendly Environments" (Chap. 3) by Ümran Topcu and Şebnem Cana Kacar. This chapter brings together planning and design elements to consider how built environments can help improve and foster well-being in children. Using the case of Istanbul, Turkey, this chapter considers the impact of rapid urbanization and the need for building child-friendly communities in cities. It provides a case of aspects to consider for transforming urban environments into those that support children's well-being, such as mobility, and involvement in planning decisions. A design proposal and process is presented for this purpose.

While rapid urbanization is a major consideration throughout many places in the world, the opposite is of concern for others. YeonKyeong Lee and Seung Jong Lee provide a view of gauging well-being in Chap. 4, "Community Well-Being and Migration Intention of Residents". Using the case of Korea, where there is deep concern with population declines, they consider impacts on overall well-being at the local level. The study examines the intention of residents to migrant away or stay within their current communities. Looking at a range of community characteristics, they consider the influences exerted on migration intention. This is particularly relevant for those places with declining population but also will be of interest in seeing how the framework of analysis was constructed for considering the influences of objective community characteristics.

"Perceived Social Support Systems for Bereaved Students in Walter Sisulu University: A Pilot Study" (Chap. 5) by Sabine Baninzi and T. Mdleleni-Bookholane is the fifth chapter. Grief is a topic that is sometimes not given full consideration, and especially in the context of quality of life and well-being. This study considers students at the University who participated in a questionnaire and scale for perceived social support. As most are aware, social relationships (which could be considered support) are critical factors influencing well-being. It is an illuminating case showing that students often do not receive support during grieving.

Next, "Community Well-Being Data Collection Methodology, the Case of Enschede, the Netherlands" (Chap. 6) by Javier Martinez and Frans van den Bosch describes the methodology for data collection in a community well-being survey. Using a community well-being survey designed by the Community Well-being Institute previously used for a district in Seoul, South Korea, this study provides an in-depth perspective of how to collect well-being data to use in the communal context.

Chapter 7, "The Relationship Between the Types of Needs Satisfaction and Subjective Well-Being", by Young Woong Kang and Seung Jong Lee seeks to clarify relationships between satisfaction type of residents' needs and subjective well-being. As with the prior chapter, it utilizes the community well-being survey framework. With data analysis, it reveals the relationship between the type of satisfaction of residents and subjective well-being. Further, the authors suggest what can serve to influence happiness after basic needs are met and provide recommendations for the direction of local government policies to foster increased community well-being.

"Shredding the Evidence: Whose Collective Impact are We Talking About?" (Chap. 8) by Geoffrey Woolcock explores the interest in the North American-informed Collective Impact (CI) approach and intentions of achieving transformative social change at both the individual and community levels. As the author explains, that in Australia "the rise of CI's visibility has emerged alongside diminishing public funding for social change initiatives, with a corresponding and somewhat belated turn to the philanthropic sector to partially meet this funding shortfall." Issues and challenges of the CI method are considered and compared with other methods for gauging social impact and change.

Chapter 9 provides an exploration of fiscal structures and residents' well-being, by Youngkyun Oh. The author uses the case of Korea to explore local financial expenditures from the perspective of accountability. It explores ways to reorganize role apportionment for community well-being and residents' involvement in financial decision-making at the local level. Looking at this from the fiscal structure perspective, the chapter provides a way to consider an important element of governance—funding and financial resources—through the lens of community well-being.

Next, we shift our attention to the aspects of community well-being that often do not receive enough attention: the arts. This chapter, "Arts and Community Well-Being" (Chap. 10), by HeeKyung Sung first begins with an exploration of a wide array of community well-being literature, and then domains or dimensions of community well-being such as individual, social, and economic well-being are discussed. Further, the notion of arts and cultural impacts within community well-being dimensions is discussed from several different perspectives. A proposed conceptual model of arts and community well-being is then presented, along with propositions that can be used to examine the relationship between arts and cultural assets and community well-being outcomes.

The volume concludes with the chapter, "Spirituality: The Missing Link of Sustainability and Happiness as a Framework for Holistic Development" (Chap. 11), by Erica Berejnoi, Rohana Ulluwishewa, Scott Cloutier, Leah Gibbons, and Susana Puga. Another topic that needs more attention in the literature, their work brings together perspectives on the interrelationship between sustainability and happiness. And while happiness promotes sustainable behaviors, sustainable behaviors likewise enhance happiness. Happiness, as it influences overall well-being is considered. Spirituality as a crucial differentiating element is proposed both as a source of happiness and sustainability, and ultimately, enhanced community well-being.

It is our sincere hope that this volume will be both inspiring and informative to those interested in learning more about community well-being applications and approaches in a variety of contexts across communities of place and interest. There is much work to be done in this varied landscape of community well-being and we encourage you to explore how to foster better understanding and application, from a variety of perspectives.

Seoul, Korea (Republic of) Youngwha Kee
Seoul, Korea (Republic of) Seung Jong Lee
West Lafayette, USA Rhonda Phillips

References

Haworth, J., & Hart, G. (2007). *Well-being: Individual, community and social perspectives*. Hampshire: Palgrave.

Kee, Y., & Nam, C. (2016). Does sense of community matter in community well-being? In Y. Kee, S.J. Lee & R. Phillips (Eds.), *Social factors and community well-being* (pp. 39–56). Dordrecht, The Netherlands: Springer. www.springer.com/us/bok/9783319299402.

Lee, S.J., Kim, Y., & Phillips, R. (2015). Exploring the intersection of community well-being and community development. In S.J. Lee, Y. Kim & Y. Phillip (Eds.), *Community well-being and community development* (pp. 1–7). Dordrecht, The Netherlands: Springer. www.springer.com/social+sciences/wellbeing+%26+quality-of-life/book/978-3-319-12420-9.

Lee, S.J., & Kim, Y. (2015). Searching for the meaning of community well-being. In S.J. Lee, Y. Kim & Y. Phillip (Eds.), *Community well-being and community development* (pp. 9–23). Dordrecht, The Netherlands: Springer.

Phillips, R., & Wong, C. (2016). Introduction. In R. Phillips & C. Wong (Eds.), *The handbook of community well-being* (pp. xxix–xxxviii). Dordrecht: Springer.

Sung, H., & Phillips, R. (2016). Conceptualizing a community well-being and theory construct. In S.J. Lee, Y. Kee & R. Phillips (Eds.), *Social factors and community well-being* (pp. 1–12). Dordrecht: Springer.

Acknowledgements

We would like to thank the National Research Foundation of Korea, funded by the Korean Government (NRF-2016S1A3A2924563), for support of research represented in several chapters of this book. We also acknowledge the International Society for Quality-of-Life Studies which provided the venue for several of these papers to be presented at the Phoenix, Arizona conference.

Contents

Editors and Contributors

About the Editors

Youngwha Kee is Professor in the Department of Lifelong Education at Soongsil University. She has served as the President of the Association of Adult and Continuing Education of Korea and Director of the Korea Institute of Local Development Education. Currently, she serves on the editorial board of Springer's Community Quality-of-Life and Well-Being book series, the *International Journal of Continuing Education and Lifelong Learning* (Hong Kong), the Lifelong Education Magazine (Taiwan), and Lifelong Education (China). Her research interests include educational gerontology, community and civic education, community well-being, community development, and governance.

Seung Jong Lee is a Professor and Dean of the Graduate School of Public Administration, Seoul National University. Previously, he served as the president of the Korean Association for Public Administration and as chief editor of several academic journals in related fields. He has frequently advised local and national governments through such positions as Chairman of the Local Government Administration Joint Evaluation Committee, Vice-Chairman of the Presidential Committee on Local District Reorganization Plans, and member of the presidential transition committee. He has not only done extensive research on citizen participation and local autonomy but has also been a strong advocate and educator in the field. He is the author of *Theories of Local Autonomy,* and *Democratic Politics and Citizen Participation.*

Rhonda Phillips, Ph.D., FAICP is a member of the College of Fellows of the American Institute of Certified Planners (FAICP). At Purdue University, she is inaugural Dean of the Honors College, and Professor, Agricultural Economics Department at Purdue University. She is author or editor of several books, including *The Handbook of Community Well-Being* (2017, Springer) and *The Handbook of Community Development, Perspectives from Across the Globe* (2018, Routledge).

She is editor of two book series, *Community Quality of Life and Well-Being*, www.springer.com/series/13761, and editor of *Community Development Research and Practice,* www.routledge.com/Community-Development-Research-and-Practice-Series/book-series/CDRP. She served as president of the International Society for Quality-of-Life Studies, www.isqols.org and on the Board of Directors for the Community Indicator Consortium, http://communityindicators.net/. Along with Seung Lee, she is co-editor of the new Springer journal, *The International Journal of Community Well-Being,* www.springer.com/social+sciences/wellbeing+&+quality-of-life/journal/42413.

Contributors

Lidia R. Arends Erasmus University Rotterdam, Rotterdam, The Netherlands

Sabi Baninzi Faculty of Humanities, Social Sciences and Law, Department of Social Work and Psychology, Walter Sisulu University, Mthatha, Eastern Cape, South Africa

Erica Berejnoi Arizona State University, Tempe, AZ, USA

Frans van den Bosch Faculty ITC—PGM, University of Twente, Enschede, The Netherlands

Scott Cloutier Arizona State University, Tempe, AZ, USA

Leah Gibbons Tempe, AZ, USA

Lena Henning Happiness Research Organisation, Dusseldorf, Germany

Sebnem Cana Kacar Bahçeşehir Üniversitesi, Kuzey Kampüsü, Mimarlık ve Tasarım Fakültesi, Abbasağa Mahallesi, Beşiktaş, İstanbul, Turkey

Young Woong Kang Graduate School of Public Administration, Seoul National University, Seoul, South Korea

Pat Lauderdale Arizona State University, Tempe, AZ, USA

Seung Jong Lee Graduate School of Public Administration, Seoul National University, Seoul, South Korea

YeonKyeong Lee Graduate School of Public Administration, Seoul National University, Seoul, South Korea

Kai Ludwigs Happiness Research Organisation, Dusseldorf, Germany

Javier Martinez Faculty ITC—PGM, University of Twente, Enschede, The Netherlands

T. Mdleleni-Bookholane Faculty of Humanities, Social Sciences and Law, Department of Social Work and Psychology, Walter Sisulu University, Mthatha, Eastern Cape, South Africa

Youngkyun Oh Humanities & Social Science College, Suwon University, Gyeonggi, South Korea

Susana Puga Tempe, AZ, USA

HeeKyung Sung Department of Recreation and Tourism Management, California State University, Northridge, CA, USA

E. Ümran Topcu Bahçeşehir Üniversitesi, Kuzey Kampüsü, Mimarlık ve Tasarım Fakültesi, Abbasağa Mahallesi, Beşiktaş, İstanbul, Turkey

Rohana Ulluwishewa Palmerston North, New Zealand

Anura Uthumange Center for Spirituality in Sustainable Business Management, Faculty of Management Studies and Commerce, University of Sri Jayewardenepura, Gangodawila, Sri Lanka

Geoffrey Woolcock Institute for Resilient Regions, University of Southern Queensland, Springfield/Toowoomba, MA, Australia

Chapter 1
Measuring Happiness—A Practical Review

Kai Ludwigs, Lena Henning and Lidia R. Arends

Abstract In times of increasing depression rates, happiness has gained interest as a goal for individuals and society instead of merely increasing gross domestic product. Unfortunately, happiness research remains a young discipline; thus, the definition of the term happiness is unclear across various disciplines, and many different measurement techniques have been developed and used thus far. This book chapter reviews different happiness definitions and ultimately selects the one used by the World Database of Happiness to then review which measurements are used and how frequently and to then evaluate their psychometric quality by reviewing published research thus far. In the end, the chapter presents a practical guideline of what a researcher should be aware of when measuring happiness.

Keywords Happiness · Measurements · World database of happiness · Happiness psychometrics

1.1 Introduction

Psychological diseases such as burnout and depression are on the rise these days. Accordingly, the World Health Organisation (WHO) forecasts that in 2030, depression will be the most common disease in high-income countries (Allianz & RWI, 2011; Mathers & Loncar, 2006). But this is not a problem that individuals must address on their own; rather, it is also of tremendous relevance for the economy. Indeed, psychological diseases already cause yearly economic costs of at least 7

K. Ludwigs (✉) · L. Henning
Happiness Research Organisation, Grafenberger Allee 342, 40235 Dusseldorf, Germany
e-mail: ludwigs@happiness-research.org

L. Henning
e-mail: info@happiness-research.org

L. R. Arends
Erasmus University Rotterdam, Rotterdam, Netherlands
e-mail: arends@fsw.eur.nl

© Springer Nature Switzerland AG 2019

Y. Kee et al. (eds.), *Perspectives on Community Well-Being*, Community Quality-of-Life and Well-Being, https://doi.org/10.1007/978-3-030-15115-7_1

billion euro, as calculated, for example, for the German population (DGPPN, 2013). The main reasons for high massive expenditures are the direct costs of therapy and indirect costs caused by general productivity loss (Allianz & RWI, 2011).

1.1.1 Beneficial Effects of Happiness

By comparison, people who live a happy and fulfilling life exhibit various positive characteristics. They are less likely to get sick, and they have a better immune system (Pressman & Cohen, 2005). Moreover, happy people tend to live longer (Danner, Snowdon, & Friesen, 2001; Diener & Chan, 2011), and states with happier citizens have lower suicide rates (Koivumaa-Honkanen, Honkanen, Koskenvuo, & Kaprio, 2003). Additionally, happiness is a crucial factor for job and general satisfaction (Judge & Watanabe, 1993), and in turn, higher job satisfaction predicts lower job turnover rates (Clark, Georgellis, & Sanfey, 1998; Frijters, 2000). Happy people also put more effort into their work and thus work harder (Judge, Thoresen, Bono, & Patton, 2001). Overall, it is thus not surprising that numerous surveys show a positive relationship between people's happiness and their productivity in different contexts (Cropanzano & Wright, 1999; Haas & Janssen, 2012; Harter, Schmidt, Asplund, & Kilham, 2010; Isen, Daubman, & Nowicki, 1987; Lyubomirsky, King & Diener, 2005; Oishi, 2012; Oswald, Proto, & Sgroi, 2009; Wright & Cropanzano, 2004; Wright & Staw, 1999). Concerning the economy, happy people are associated with increased health, effort and innovative actions, which ultimately leads to better long-term economic welfare. But the list of benefits that happy people may bring continues. In fact, such people are more sociable (George, 1991), more engaged in prosocial behaviours (Cunningham, Steinberg, & Grev, 1980; Isen, 1970), more likely to volunteer more often (Thoits & Hewitt, 2001), more likely to donate (Priller & Schupp, 2011) and more likely to give more money to charities (Aknin, Sandstrom, Dunn, & Norton, 2011). Therefore, happy people influence not only economic factors positively but also social progress.

Against this background, it is completely rational and understandable that some nations have worked on implementing (e.g., Great Britain, England's Prime Minister David Cameron: Cameron, 2006; Stratton, 2010; White, 2007; France, Former President Nicolas Sarcozy: Jolly, 2009; Stiglitz, Sen, & Fitoussi, 2009) or have clearly announced and prioritized (Bhutan, King Jigme Singye Wangchuck: Pfaff, 2011; Priesner 1999) a more intense focus on happiness when measuring economic performance and social progress. Accordingly, the European Commission, European Parliament, Club of Rome, OECD, and WWF discussed in 2007 how to improve progress and conditions of societies differently from merely focusing on economic factors (Commission of the European Communities, 2009). Many researchers have also intensely discussed this topic in the scientific community (Diener, 2000, 2012; Diener & Seligman, 2004; Di Tella & MacCulloch, 2008; Dolan & White, 2007; Frey & Stutzer, 2002; Kahneman & Krueger, 2006; Kahneman, Krueger, Schkade, Schwarz, & Stone, 2004a; MacKerron, 2012).

It can be concluded that pursuing a happier society, that is, achieving a higher level of happiness for everyone (Veenhoven, 2010), seems to be worthwhile. But the following question remains: what can we do to reach this goal? To answer this question, we need to investigate the important factors and their interrelations that determine happiness. However, to be able to do so, some premises need to be met: (i) We need to know what we mean by happiness. Thus, we need a clear definition of this construct. (ii) We need measures that capture the defined concept of happiness as valid and as feasible as possible. Consequently, we need to investigate existing measures in terms of their (psychometric) quality and their applicability in various situations (e.g., research questions; populations). By doing so, we can determine the best way to assess happiness depending on the current context. The current book chapter aims to contribute to meeting these 2 premises in future studies.

1.2 Definition of Happiness

For a long time, scholars have immensely engaged with the topic of happiness and the pursuit thereof. Ancient philosophy was concerned with the question of what is a good life, which was typically considered a morally good life denoted with the term happiness. For instance, Aristotle described striving for happiness as the most important of all goals and as the goal of life itself, as articulated in the following quotation: "Happiness is the meaning and the purpose of life, the whole aim and end of human existence" (as cited in: Bacon, Brophy, Mguni, Mulgan, & Shandro, 2010, p. 10). Other thinkers of ancient times, such as the Indian intellectual Dhammapada or philosophers from Confucianism, Taoism, and Buddhism (Judge & Kammeyer-Mueller, 2011; Lu, 2001), were also concerned with this question. In the Middle Ages, Thomas Aquinas stated that happiness was "the ultimate goal of the rational being" (Judge & Kammeyer-Mueller, 2011, p. 31) and therewith underlined the importance of striving for happiness. Finally, the American Declaration of Independence (1776) names the pursuit of happiness as one of the unalienable rights besides life and liberty and thus as one of the ultimate rights and goals of every human being. This follows the idea of Jeremy Bentham, who stated in his doctrine: "Create all the happiness you are able to create; remove all the misery you are able to remove" (as cited in: Layard, 2005, p. 235).

1.2.1 Divergent Use of the Word

In sum, talking about happiness is not new at all, but the meaning of the word might have changed somewhat. However, research in this field remains very young and has particularly expanded since the 1990s (MacKerron, 2012; OECD, 2013). This is also reflected in the relatively recent launch of the *Journal of Happiness Studies,* which has published papers on happiness since 2000 (Journal of Happiness Studies, 2016).

As the discipline is so young, final agreement about the relevant terminology and definitions is currently lacking. In Easterlin (2003) posited that for him, happiness could be equated with utility, well-being, life satisfaction, and welfare. Other researchers have added additional terms that have often been used synonymously with happiness, such as "pleasure, life satisfaction, positive emotions, a meaningful life, or a feeling of contentment" (Diener, Scollon, & Lucas, 2003, p. 188). In their paper, Diener, Scollon, & Lucas (2003) use happiness and subjective well-being (SWB) interchangeably, and in accordance such usage, Seligman & Csikszentmihalyi (2000) stated that the term SWB is actually just "a more scientific-sounding term for what people usually mean by happiness" (p. 9; also cp. Diener, 2000, p. 24).

1.2.2 Need for a Clear Definition

Overall, this inconsistency in terminology can only cause confusion. To be clear in meaning in this book chapter, we will exclusively rely on the term happiness throughout to be consistent with the general tone of the entire book. In addition, we prefer the term happiness because we perceive it to be more easy-going and understandable for all readers. Concerning the abovementioned challenge in definition, it must be said that there is no consensus between researchers in their different disciplines for a common definition of happiness (cp. Lu, 2001; Veenhoven, 1984, 2010). Here, a definition for happiness is presented with the aim of (i) integrating the most common definition but also (ii) differentiating the adopted definition from definitions that are relatively vague and probably too broad to capture happiness alone. This definition serves as a basis for the following selection and review of happiness measures. By choosing such a clear concept of happiness, we can assure that the measure selection contains only measures that really fit this definition.

1.2.3 What Happiness Means from Our Point of View

In general, research and survey literature has often emphasized two aspects related to happiness (Busseri & Sadava, 2011; Clark & Senik, 2011; Diener, 2000; Diener, Scollon, & Lucas, 2003; Diener, Suh, Lucas, & Smith, 1999; Dolan & White, 2007; Lucas, Diener, & Suh, 1996; OECD, 2013; Stiglitz et al., 2009): (1) the emotional or affective aspect ("a person's feelings or emotional states, typically measured with reference to a particular point in time": OECD, 2013, p. 10) and (2) the rational, cognitive or evaluative aspect ("a reflective assessment on a person's life or some specific aspect of it": OECD, 2013, p. 10). On the one hand, some happiness definitions especially concentrate on the emotional aspect, as with the one of Bradburn (1969, p. 9), who referred to happiness as the "resultant of the individual's position on two independent dimensions – one of positive affect and the other of negative affect." Another well-known definition is the one of Goldings, who stated in (1954, p. 31) that happiness for him "embraces feelings of elation, contentment, satisfaction, and pleasure at the positive pole and feelings of depression, discontent, and unpleasure at the negative pole."

Further, affect-focused happiness definitions can also be found in Flügel (1925), Fordyce (1977) and Wessman and Ricks (1966). On the other hand, happiness definitions pay particularly attention to the evaluative aspect. Lemon, Bengtson, & Peterson (1972, p. 513), for example, referred to happiness as "the degree to which one is presently content or pleased with his general life situation," whereas Tatarkiewicz (1966, p. 1) merely briefly stated that happiness can be equated with "satisfaction with one's life as a whole." Another, evaluation-focused happiness definition can, for instance, be found in Michalos (1980). In addition to these either affect- or evaluation-focused happiness definitions, some definitions do not have a clear emphasis and combine both aspects instead. One exemplary and well-noticed definition comes from Diener, who wrote in (2000, p. 34) that happiness for him means "people's cognitive and affective evaluations of their lives" (adapted versions can be found in Diener, 2012; Diener, Scollon, & Lucas, 2003; Diener et al., 1999). Another frequently cited definition of happiness was launched by the OECD (2013, p. 29), which considers happiness to refer to "Good mental states, including all of the various evaluations, positive and negative, that people make of their lives, and the affective reactions of people to their experiences." Further happiness definitions have also been proposed by Busseri and Sadava (2011), Dolan and White (2007) and Sumner (1996).

In sum, all the suggested happiness definitions deal with either feelings or cognitions or combine them both. But none of them assumes the affective and cognitive aspect as components of or views on happiness. In contrast to these previous definitions, our happiness definition does exactly this. Although our approach differs from previous ones in this manner, it is nevertheless generally aligned with the vast majority of literature using an affective and/or cognitive aspect in the definition of happiness (see above for single definitions). Thus, we define *Overall Happiness* as "the overall enjoyment of one's life as-a-whole" (Veenhoven, 2010, p. 611; cp. Veenhoven, 1984, 1991, 1994, 1997, 2008).

This general evaluation is then "based on both affective and cognitive appraisals of life" (Veenhoven, 2010, p. 611, cp. Veenhoven, 1984) or a "dual evaluation system" (Veenhoven, 2000, p. 14). The *Affective Happiness Component* of this system is meant to evaluate "the degree to which the various affects a person experiences are pleasant; in other words: how well he usually feels" (Veenhoven, 1991, p. 10; cp. Veenhoven, 1984, 2010). The *Cognitive Happiness Component* of this system is then meant to evaluate "the degree to which an individual perceives his aspirations to have been met. In other words: to what extent one perceives oneself to have got what one wants in life" (Veenhoven, 1991, p. 10; cp. Veenhoven, 1984, 2010). Although this dual evaluation system composes the overall happiness evaluation, the latter should be considered separately in surveys. Given this idea, the construct of happiness should in sum be considered "a kind of trinity" (Veenhoven, 1984, p. 28). This approach makes sense when considering the following examples (derived from Veenhoven, 1984, p. 32), in which the calculation of overall happiness using only individuals' affective and cognitive judgments is rather unclear: (i) someone is more or less dissatisfied with what he/she has achieved in life but nevertheless feels tremendously good; (ii) someone obtained everything he/she wanted but nevertheless feels downhearted. Although research results suggest that affective aspects usually influence overall life evaluations more than cognitive ones (Schwarz & Strack, 1991; Veenhoven, 1997, 2000, 2010), we do not know the exact weighting of the factors. Besides this content-related reason, pragmatics play a role when favouring an additional overall happiness evaluation in surveys, as most researchers use overall happiness indicators in their studies (Veenhoven, 1984).

1.2.4 What Happiness Does not Mean from Our Point of View

To create a clear definition of our happiness construct, it does make sense to define not only what happiness is but also what happiness is not in our understanding. We already fulfilled the first aspect in discussing what we exactly understand by the term happiness. To meet the second aspect, we first collected conditions that are regularly associated with the word happiness today and arranged them in a 2 × 2 matrix (Veenhoven, 2000, 2008, 2010; see Table 1.1). As Table 1.1 shows, happiness in our understanding is something that is judged in "the eye of the beholder" (Veenhoven, 2010, p. 608) and that concerns actual life (not only pre-conditions for a happy life).

Similarly, Table 1.2 shows the relation of our happiness definition with other kinds of satisfaction that can be expressed by persons. In accordance with this visualization, happiness in our understanding concerns life evaluations that are not momentary and thus fleeting—but rather enduring (Veenhoven, 1997). Additionally, our happiness concept entails an evaluation focusing on overall life, not single life aspects, such as work and marriage (Veenhoven, 1984, 1997). Yet, studies have investigated the contribution of life domains to overall happiness. For example, Van Praag, Frijters, & Ferrer-i-Carbonell (2003) found that finance, health, and job satisfaction influence overall happiness in individuals to the highest extent. However, remarkably, the authors included only 6 life domains in their analysis. Consequently, they may not

Table 1.1 Conditions regularly associated with the word happiness today, classified into a 2 × 2 matrix

	Outside the person	Inside the person
Possibilities	Liveability of the environment	Life-ability
Outcomes	Utility of life	*Happiness*

Notes Adapted from Veenhoven (2010, p. 608). Closer explanation of the terms used (p. 608): *Liveability of the Environment* = "good living conditions"; *Life-ability* = extent to which the person is "equipped to cope with the problems of life"; *Utility of life* = "a good life must be good for something more than itself", e.g., for "ecological preservation or cultural development"; *Happiness* = as we understand and defined it above

Table 1.2 Various kinds of satisfaction that can be expressed by persons, classified into a 2 × 2 matrix

	Passing	Enduring
Part of life	Pleasure	Part happiness
Life as a whole	Peak experience	*Happiness*

Note Adapted from Veenhoven (2010, p. 609). Closer explanation of the terms used (p. 609): *Pleasure* = "can be sensoric, such as a glass of good wine, or mental, such as the reading of this text"; *Part happiness* = "can concern a domain of life, such as working-life, and an aspect of life, such as its variety"; *Peak experience* = "intense and oceanic" experience, also known as "enlightenment"; *Happiness* = as we understand and defined it above

cover all relevant life domains. Accordingly, Dolan and White (2007) have criticized that how all the different life domains relatively contribute to overall happiness remains unclear today. But even if a researcher considered all important life domains, he still would not be able to calculate a precise overall happiness score because the importance weighting of every life domain for overall happiness has been shown to be highly individual (Diener, Lucas, Oishi, & Suh, 2002; Diener, Scollon, & Lucas, 2003). Thus, it currently remains unclear (i) which domains should be of relevance for overall happiness and (ii) how an overall happiness score can be gained from domain evaluation judgments. Life domains are therefore unsuitable as indicators for overall happiness in a precise happiness definition. Nevertheless, they can deliver valuable insights for researchers who are especially interested in particular life domains. These indicators could then even prove more meaningful than global judgments of happiness in such cases (see also Diener, Scollon, & Lucas, 2003 for this opinion).

Another topic that needs to be discussed and distinguished from our happiness concept is *eudaimonia*. The term was originally created by Aristotle, who is today considered "the father" (Bruni, 2010, p. 391) of the eudaimonian happiness approach. According to him, eudaimonia can be equated with happiness. Similarly, "happiness is the final, or ultimate, end of life: [It] is the 'highest good' for the human being" (Bruni, 2010, p. 392). It is characterized as "something like flourishing human living, a kind of living that is active, inclusive of all that has intrinsic value, and complete, meaning lacking in nothing that would make it richer or better" (Nussbaum, 2005, p. 171). Consequently, happiness can be reached by practicing virtues not in an instrumental way but in an intrinsically motivated way, where virtues are internalized and thus perceived as important and good to follow (*Aristotle's happiness paradox*; Bruni, 2010). Against this philosophical background, some researchers have suggested that not only affective and cognitive aspects but also eudaimonian aspects should be considered when defining happiness (e.g., Clark & Senik, 2011; Diener et al., 2010; Huppert et al., 2009; OECD, 2013; Ryan & Deci, 2001). Such aspects are meant to add individual judgments about the perceived degree "of meaning and purpose in life, or [of] good psychological functioning" (OECD, 2013, p. 10).

In general, the importance of considering the concept of eudaimonia in a definition of happiness should be discussed in the future. However, to date, little research has confirmed its relevance for a definition of happiness, in addition to the affective and cognitive components. Instead, current research literature indicates that eudaimonia should be considered a moderating or influencing factor with respect to actual happiness rather than a clear component of happiness itself. For example, the OECD (2013) admits that the eudaimonian view on happiness brings a "more instrumental focus" (p. 32) with it than the perspective on affective and cognitive components. Further evidence for this point of view can be derived from investigations conducted in the context of *Self-Determination Theory* (SDT; Ryan & Deci 2000). According to this theory, three factors that are associated with self-realization or eudaimonia (autonomy, competence, and relatedness) basically contribute to an individual's degree of happiness (Ryan & Deci 2000, 2001). In addition to this content-related argumentation, further findings on the reliability and validity of eudaimonic measures are required (Dolan, Peasgood, & White, 2006; OECD, 2013) to be able to guarantee high psychometric quality when assessing eudaimonia in individuals.

In sum, no definition of happiness that is generally accepted currently exists. Thus, a concept that is as precise as possible and that fits with most common literature on affective and/or cognitive aspects of happiness is presented here. In our view, Overall Happiness can be equated with "the overall enjoyment of one's life as-a-whole" (Veenhoven, 2010, p. 611; cp. Veenhoven, 1984, 1991, 1994, 1997, 2008). Further, the Affective Happiness Component evaluates "the degree to which the various affects a person experiences are pleasant; in other words: how well he usually feels" (Veenhoven, 1991, p. 10; cp. Veenhoven, 1984, 2010). By contrast, the Cognitive Happiness Component covers "the degree to which an individual perceives his aspirations to have been met. In other words: to what extent one perceives oneself to have got what one wants in life" (Veenhoven, 1991, p. 10; cp. Veenhoven, 1984, 2010). These definitions now serve as a basis for our selection of appropriate happiness measures to investigate them in terms of quality and applicability.

Measures of Happiness

The World Database of Happiness (WDOH; Veenhoven, 2016a) constitutes a library that fairly exhaustingly collects publications on happiness. In addition, it offers distributional and correlational findings that are calculated by the author and his co-workers themselves. In the context of this article, the WDOH is particularly helpful because it also offers a collection of happiness measures that are based on the above-mentioned happiness definition (Veenhoven, 2016b). Currently,[1] 2,118 measures are listed, and most are self-reports on single questions (1,516 measures, equalling 71.58%).

Classification

All accepted measures in the WDOH are classified by the (i) kind of happiness addressed, (ii) time frame, (iii) measure technique, and (iv) scaling. Each classification category is described in the following, based on Veenhoven (2015). Illustrative item examples are also given.

[1]As assessed on January 31st, 2017.

The Kind of Happiness Addressed

As stated above, we assume that three components should be measured to capture happiness: Overall Happiness, the Affective Happiness Component and the Cognitive Happiness Component. In accordance with this view, all measures are assigned to one of these categories. For measures either that are ambiguous or that can definitely be classified to various categories, another fourth category is available (*Mixed Measures*).

Examples:

- Overall Happiness: "How do you feel about your life as a whole…?"
  - Rating: 7-point scale: 1: terrible, 2: unhappy, 3: mostly dissatisfied, 4: mixed, 5: mostly satisfied, 6: pleased, 7: delighted
  - Reference: Andrews and Withey (1976).
- Affective Happiness Component: "How is your mood these days…?"
  - Rating: 4-point scale: 1: not good almost all the time, 4: very good all the time
  - Reference: Levy and Guttman (1975).
- Cognitive Happiness Component: "How do you feel about what you are accomplishing in life…?"
  - Rating: 7-point scale: 1: completely dissatisfied, 2: very dissatisfied, 3: dissatisfied, 4: satisfied-dissatisfied, 5: satisfied, 6: very satisfied, 7: completely satisfied
  - Reference: Buttel and Martinson (1977).
- Mixed Measures: "How many days in the previous week did you feel happy?"
  - Rating: 8-point scale: 0: none, 7: all
  - Reference: Simon and Nath (2004).

Time Frame

This category expresses the period of happiness addressed. The following time frames are included in the WDOH:

- Momentary, Now
- Last Instant
- Last Hour
- Last Part of the Day
- Last Day
- Yesterday
- Last Week
- Last Month, Last Few Weeks
- Last Quarter

- Last Year
- Last Years
- Over Lifetime
- Currently (Presently, Today, These Days)
- Generally
- Hitherto
- Since Event
- Various Time Frames (in Case of Mixed Measures)
- Time Frame Unspecified
- Time Frame Not Reported.

Examples:

- Momentary, Now: "How are you feeling now…?"
  - Rating: 5-point scale: 1: very poor, 2: poor, 3: neither good nor poor, 4: good, 5: very good
  - Reference: Ventegodt (1995).
- Yesterday: "Overall, how happy did you feel yesterday?"
  - Rating: 11-point scale: 0: not at all, 10: completely
  - Reference: Office for National Statistics (2012).
- Last Year: "Generally, how happy have you been with your personal life during the past 12 months?"
  - Rating: 5-point scale: 1: unhappy most of the time, 2: sometimes fairly unhappy, 3: generally satisfied, pleased, 4: very happy most of the time, 5: extremely happy
  - Reference: Else-Quest, Hyde, and DeLamater (2005).
- Currently (Presently, Today, These Days): "All things considered, how would you describe yourself these days? Would you say you are…?"
  - Rating: 3-point scale: 1: not too happy, 2: fairly happy, 3: very happy
  - Reference: Kantor, Milton, and Ernst (1978).

Measurement Technique

Here, the WDOH mainly distinguishes between self-reports on single or multiple closed questions, open questions or ego-documents (e.g., diaries) and ratings by others, such as clinicians, peers, own family or teachers.

Examples:

- Self-Report: "In thinking over the past year, indicate how elated or depressed, happy or unhappy you have felt in the last year?"
  - Rating: 10-point scale: 1: Utter depression and gloom. Completely down. All is black and leaden. Wish it were all over. 2: Tremendously depressed. Feeling

terrible, really miserable, "just awful". 3: Depressed and feeling very low. Definitely "blue". 4: Spirits low and somewhat "blue". 5: Feeling a little bit low. Just so-so. 6: Feeling pretty good, "OK". 7: Feeling very good and cheerful. 8: Elated and in high spirits. 9: Very elated and in very high spirits. Tremendous delight and buoyancy. 10: Complete elation, rapturous joy and soaring ecstasy.
  - Reference: Constantinople (1967).

- Rating by Others: "Overall how does your child usually feel?"
  - Rating: 7-point smiley scale: from sad face to happy face
  - Reference: Holder, Coleman, and Wallace (2010).

Scaling

Answers to questions can be given on different scales. The WDOH differentiates between four different scale-type categories. Verbal scales have each response option labelled, whereas numerical scales have only extremes defined. Graphical scales can be a scale with smiley faces, a ladder, a mountain or a thermometer, and the last category, miscellaneous scales, includes scales that cannot be classified among the former ones, such as the percentage of time being happy.

Examples:

- Verbal Scales: "How do you feel about your life as a whole…?"
  - Rating: 7-point scale: 1: terrible, 2: unhappy, 3: mostly dissatisfied, 4: mixed, 5: mostly satisfied, 6: pleased, 7: delighted
  - Reference: Andrews and Withey (1976).
- Numerical Scales: "How is your mood these days…?"
  - Rating: 4-point scale: 1: not good almost all the time, 4: very good all the time
  - Reference: Levy and Guttman (1975).
- Graphical Scales: "Overall how does your child usually feel?"
  - Rating: 7-point smiley scale: from sad face to happy face
  - Reference: Holder, Coleman, and Wallace (2010).
- Miscellaneous Scales:
  - A: "What percentage of time that you were awake today did you feel happy?"
  - B: "What percentage did you feel unhappy?"
  - C: "What percentage did you feel neither happy nor unhappy?"
    Rating: Percentages should in total sum up to 100%
    Reference: Kammann and Flett (1983).

Table 1.3 reports how often each sub-category is listed in the WDOH in relation to specific population groups.

Table 1.3 Number of available studies for all classification categories, as listed in the WDOH*

WDOH category	Frequency of studies
(i) Kind of happiness addressed	
Overall happiness	459
Affective happiness component	114
Cognitive happiness component	1,243
Mixed measures	311
(ii) Time frame	
Momentary, now	47
Last instant	50
Last hour	8
Last part of the day	7
Last day	41
Yesterday	51
Last week	100
Last month, last few weeks	115
Last quarter	14
Last year	46
Last years	5
Over lifetime	3
Currently (presently, today, these days)	532
Generally	310
Hitherto	46
Since event	9
Various time frames (in case of mixed measures)	75
Time frame unspecified	498
Time frame not reported	171
(iii) Measure technique	
Self-report	1,982
Rating by others	141
(iv) Scaling	
Verbal scales	1,288
Numerical scales	556
Graphical scales	139
Miscellaneous scales	145

*As assessed on January 31st, 2017

Psychometric Considerations

In happiness research, there has been a long-lasting debate about the extent to which the happiness construct can be reliably and validly measured (cp. Kahneman, 1994; MacKerron, 2012; Veenhoven, 1984, 2010). But research in this field today generally underlines the point of view that happiness can be reliably and validly measured (e.g., Diener, Suh, & Oishi, 1997; Diener et al., 1999; Judge & Kammeyer-Mueller, 2011; Kahneman, 1994; Kahneman & Krueger, 2006; MacKerron, 2012; Veenhoven, 2010). Test-retest reliability, for example, has been demonstrated over the course of various time frames (Bradburn, 1969; Bradburn & Caplovitz, 1965; Diener & Larsen, 1984; Diener et al., 2010; Fujita & Diener, 2005; Krueger & Schkade, 2008; Lepper, 1998; Lucas & Donnellan, 2012; Michalos & Kahlke, 2010; Watson, Clark, & Tellegen, 1988). In addition, various findings show the validity of happiness measures. For instance, positive correlations between self-rated happiness scores and happiness ratings delivered by significant others (such as friends and family: Lepper, 1998; Sandvik, Diener, & Seidlitz, 1993; Schneider & Schimmack, 2009), happiness ratings given by interviewers (Pavot & Diener, 1993), the frequency of smiling when individuals interact in a social context (Fernández-Dols & Ruiz-Belda, 1995), more left than right superior frontal cortex activity (Urry et al., 2004) and lower cortisol rates and lower heart rates (Steptoe, Wardle, & Marmot, 2005) demonstrate the convergent validity of happiness measures. Further, the discriminant validity of happiness measures has been shown by the low correlation between self-rated happiness scores and optimism (Lucas, Diener, & Suh, 1996). Further results showing a positive correlation between self-rated happiness scores and specific life events (e.g., marriage) but a negative correlation between self-rated happiness scores and unemployment (Diener, 2012; Diener, Lucas & Scollon, 2006; Winkelmann & Winkelmann, 1998) demonstrate the criteria validity of happiness measures. Such evidence is further supported by positive correlations between self-rated happiness scores and level of income (Sacks, Stevenson, & Wolfers, 2010), life circumstances (e.g., health status and social contact; Dolan, Peasgood & White, 2008) and daily activities (Kahneman & Krueger, 2006). In addition, low non-response rates for happiness indicators demonstrate the face validity of happiness measures (Kahneman & Krueger, 2006; Rässler & Riphahn, 2006).

Nevertheless, the WDOH has indicated that many measures are currently available to assess individuals' happiness. The high number of measures implies quality differences in terms of psychometrics (e.g., reliability, validity) and applicability in different contexts. The strengths and weaknesses of these happiness measures are introduced in the following.

Differences in Time Frames

A few years ago, Dolan et al. (2006) noted that many happiness measures hardly use exact time frames but instead ask about the respondent's life in general. Nevertheless, given the elaborated classification of happiness measures in the WDOH in combination with corresponding practical research activities, this statement needs to be rejected. In fact, the WDOH presently[2] lists numerous measures that use different frames. For example, 531 measures incorporate wording such as "currently (today, these days, presently)", 115 measures use wording such as "last month, last few weeks", 100 measures refer to the "last week", and 51 measures refer to "yesterday". Against this background, the question arises how respondents react to various time frames and then how they ultimately form their happiness judgments. With respect to the time frame currently (today, these days, presently), for instance, how past and future happiness and associated factors influence happiness questions containing this time frame remains unclear (MacKerron, 2012). Research conducted by Watson and colleagues (1988) has shown that people tend to answer similar questions under different time frame conditions slightly differently. In particular, the mean scores of the positive and negative affect subscales of their happiness measure increased with a lengthened time frame, indicating growing positive and negative affect. Given that respondents were to estimate the extent of a specific type of affect in, e.g., the last few weeks, the results seem reasonable. Indeed, as the time frame increases, the probability of experiencing a specific type of affect also rises.

But what are the implications of the use of different time frames in happiness measures for psychometric quality? Generally, research on this relevant topic seems to be scarce (MacKerron, 2012), especially concerning validity issues. However, some important findings are available. Watson et al. (1988) found internal consistency to be unaffected by six variants of time frame. In contrast, test-retest reliability tended to increase with a larger time frame. According to the authors, the higher stability with larger time frames resulted from the respondents' approach of aggregating the types of affects they experienced on several occasions. By contrast, actual affect is more susceptible to change (Pavot & Diener, 1993); thus the stability is lower when it is assessed again at a later point in time. From a theoretical perspective, Pressman and Cohen (2005) argued that shorter time frames induce individuals to assess state happiness, whereas longer time frames induce them to assess trait happiness. As a main characteristic of traits consist of their relative stability over time, this statement provides a further explanation for the higher test-retest reliability when more extended time frames are used.

In sum, different time frames in similar questions seem to evoke varying response patterns. However, respondents' answers on not only questions with larger time frames but also on questions with shorter time frames show significant test-retest reliability (Watson et al., 1988). Thus, it currently seems reasonable to utilize happiness measures with various time frames.

Differences in Number of Items: Single-Item Measures Versus Multiple-Item Measures

According to the WDOH, the majority of current[3] happiness measures use just a single item (71.58% of 2,118 measures in total). This finding is in line with the claim of several authors that such measures seems to be the standard in (large-scale)

[2] As assessed on January 31st, 2017.

[3] As assessed on January 31st, 2017.

surveys (Clark & Senik, 2011; Diener et al., 1999; Huppert et al., 2009). Accordingly, Dolan and colleagues (2006) have underlined the quality of such measures in stating that a single item already makes it possible to identify differences in happiness among "those who are employed versus unemployed, single versus living with a partner, those who live in a state with good versus poor quality of governance, and so on" (p. 70). Test-retest reliability usually lies between 0.40 and 0.74 (Krueger & Schkade, 2008; Lepper, 1998; Lucas & Donnellan, 2012; Michalos & Kahlke, 2010). The correlation of two frequently used single-item measures, for instance, is 0.75 (Bjørnskov, 2010), indicating a degree of convergent validity. Nevertheless, measures that combine multiple items to capture happiness have better validity (Lucas et al., 1996) and test-retest reliability (range = 0.50–0.83: Diener et al., 2010; Krueger & Schkade, 2008; Lepper, 1998; Lucas et al., 1996; Michalos & Kahlke, 2010). Additionally, correlations between single-item measures and multiple-item measures are not perfect (i.e., not equal to 1.0; Diener, Nickerson, Lucas, & Sandvik, 2002; Pavot & Diener, 1993), indicating that both kinds of measures do not completely capture the same construct. Consequently, it is not surprising that discussion about how to deal with the standard procedure of using only single items when measuring happiness is ongoing (Clark & Senik, 2011).

A first challenge that needs to be addressed when using single-item measures is methodological. Because respondents might understand the question differently (MacKerron, 2012) and because preceding items are prone to influence answers to the relevant happiness question (Huppert et al., 2009; Schwarz & Strack, 1999), there is a high probability of measurement error. In contrast, multiple-item measures contribute to reducing this type of error (MacKerron, 2012; Schneider & Schimmack, 2009), and thus, they enhance reliability by aggregating responses to numerous items (Krueger & Schkade, 2008). Higher reliability should thus positively influence validity. Schneider and Schimmack (2009) found evidence for this statement: in their happiness study, correlations between self-ratings and ratings by others were shown to be higher when multiple items were used instead of single items.

The second challenge with single-item happiness measures relates to theoretical concerns. In 2012, MacKerron wondered: "Is SWB reducible to a single dimension, and thus is it meaningful to ask – as single-item SWB questions often do – for a global evaluation of happiness, wellbeing, or satisfaction with life?" (p. 8). Following the abovementioned definition of happiness that assumes the existence of two distinct components (affective vs. cognitive), this question needs to be answered with "no". The reason is that such a two-dimensional construct cannot be covered by asking only a single question. To actually get information on both components, it is necessary to assess them separately. Consequently, using a multiple-item measure broadens the "breadth of coverage" (Diener et al., 2003, p. 208) of the happiness construct and thus captures it more validly. A few years ago, similar concerns arose in terms of covering affect completely. Today, the approach of investigating negative and positive affect separately from each other, as they seem to be distinct parts of overall affect, is widely accepted (e.g., Bradburn, 1969; Busseri & Sadava, 2011; Diener et al., 2010).

In sum, from a psychometric and a theoretical point of view, multiple-item measures for assessing happiness are to be favourable to single-item measures. Nevertheless, the psychometric quality of single-item measures is nevertheless sufficient for them to be used in surveys without a guilty conscience (Diener et al., 2003; Larsen, Diener, & Emmons, 1985). The applicability section below will discuss profound reasons why it may be sometimes beneficial to use a less reliable but quicker assessment of respondents' happiness and thus to use single-item happiness measures.

Differences in Measurement Technique: Self-report Versus Rating by Others?

Overall, happiness measures today are primarily based on self-reports (Diener, 2012). This finding is also supported by the WDOH, which indicates that there are currently 1,982 self-report measures but only 141 measures containing ratings by others.[4] However, experts have repeatedly noted the many weaknesses of self-reports (Diener, Suh, & Oishi, 1997). Indeed, they are affected by "information that is salient at the time of the judgment" (Diener et al., 2003, p. 196), as most happiness questions are rather complex to respond to and thus facilitate the use of heuristics (Schwarz & Strack, 1991). One type of information that seems to be used quite often to generate happiness judgements is current mood (Diener et al., 2003; Kahneman & Krueger, 2006; Schwarz, 1988; Schwarz & Strack, 1991), which can be influenced by the immediate context, such as the weather (Schwarz & Clore, 1983), the pleasantness of the room (Schwarz, Strack, Kommer, & Wagner, 1987) and the success of one's national team when watching a soccer championship game (Schwarz et al., 1987). By contrast, contradictory evidence indicates that temporary moods influence happiness ratings only marginally, especially in comparison with longer-term influences (Eid & Diener, 1999). The influence of current mood on happiness judgments is also dependent on culture (Suh, Diener, Oishi, & Triandis, 1998). Indeed, respondents of individualistic-oriented cultures tend to particularly focus on their emotions as a reference for their happiness judgments, whereas respondents of collectivistic-oriented cultures use their emotions and cognition equally. Thus, the latter individuals are also oriented towards what significant others might think of the appropriateness of their current life. Besides possible mood influences, researchers have also noted the high potential for social desirability bias in happiness self-reports (Diener, 2000; Sandvik, Diener, & Seidlitz, 1993; Schwarz & Strack, 1991), and this phenomenon has been found to be dependent on the situation. For instance, in his meta-analytic approach, Smith (1979) showed that respondents reported higher well-being when interviewed face-to-face versus when assessed via mail survey. Consequently, avoiding personal contact in rating happiness can result in more honest judgments. Yet, some researchers have also obtained happiness judgments that were not contaminated by social desirability (Diener, Sandvik, Pavot, & Gallagher, 1991)—or at least not affected by social desirability to a substantial degree (Lepper, 1998). Another bias that can arise with self-reports results from placement or order effects, where the preceding questions may influence the following happiness question, e.g., by evoking specific feelings (Bjørnskov, 2010; Schwarz & Strack, 1991). Consequently, happiness questions should be asked at the very beginning of surveys to minimize this bias

[4]As assessed on January 31st, 2017.

(Graham, 2005). A further challenge for happiness self-reports concerns individual response styles. For instance, individuals may favour high numbers in rating scales (Diener et al., 2003).

In sum, to date, research has provided inconsistent information about the potential of various biases in self-reports. Nevertheless, the results suggest that cautious should be used with self-reports, as they are probably not free of unwanted influences. On the other hand, research evidence strictly supports the use of self-reports in surveys. For instance, based on test-retest reliability, there is substantial stability in happiness ratings from self-reports ($r = 0.40$–0.83: Diener et al., 2010; Krueger & Schkade, 2008; Lepper, 1998; Lucas & Donnellan, 2012; Lucas et al., 1996; Michalos & Kahlke, 2010). Furthermore, in calculating the relative percentage of measurement errors in happiness judgements, Ehrhardt, Saris, and Veenhoven (2000) found that a bias existed, but this bias diminished over the course of repeated surveys because of habituation processes and constant salient information that was used to make every judgment (Diener et al., 2003). Thus, particularly when asked several times over a longer time frame, people are capable of producing relatively stable self-reports. Accordingly, high correlations between self-ratings and ratings by others (Lepper, 1998; Pavot & Diener, 1993; Sandvik et al., 1993; Schneider & Schimmack, 2009) indicate that self-ratings cannot be so influenced by current mood or other circumstances (Lepper, 1998) to render them useless in happiness research. These findings have led several researchers to conclude that happiness can be measured by individual self-reports without a guilty conscience (Sandvik et al., 1993; Veenhoven, 2010). However, the above-described high correlations between self-ratings and ratings by others also underline the validity of ratings by others. For instance, it has been shown that raters who do not know the person to judge are able to precisely define his/her primary emotion at a specific point in time (Diener et al., 1999). Nevertheless, it should be noted that significant others, such family members or close friends, are not the person (or the "target") themselves who is actually judged. Thus, such a judgement "likely relies upon what the target has spoken, on how the target behaves, and on the expressions made by the target. This judgment made by a close significant other is likely a cumulative estimate of the verbal messages heard and the nonverbal expressions observed. A significant other likely has an abundant amount of information upon which to rely for such a judgment […]" (Lepper, 1998, p. 368). However, as happiness is defined as "an attitude towards one's life" (Veenhoven, 1984, p.39), scholars have criticized that such an abstract construct can hardly be observed by others and that self-ratings instead should be favoured (Veenhoven, 1984). At this point, it can be argued that close friends of the target can judge the target's happiness appropriately because close friends usually talk to each other honestly and mutually share their current feelings. Furthermore, exhibited non-verbal emotional signals may deliver important emotional information to significant others. Such signals are difficult to hide (Sandvik et al., 1993) and are thus less prone to conscious distortion by the respondent. Additionally, external ratings by experts or clinicians have the vast advantage over self-reports and ratings by significant others in that they are the most objective of these alternatives (Diener et al., 2003).

Overall, although self-reports seem to deliver meaningful information about the respondent's happiness, it may be beneficial to include additional measures with their own strengths to get a more detailed understanding of the happiness construct (Diener, 2000, 2012; Diener et al., 1997, 2003; Krueger & Schkade, 2008; Pavot & Diener, 1993; Sandvik et al., 1993). These additional measures can then compensate for some weaknesses of self-reports (Diener et al., 1997). Such a multi-measurement approach seems to be path breaking since the use of such an approach has already led to deviations from previous study results obtained from self-reports (Diener, 2012). In such an approach, however, the above-discussed ratings by others do not represent the only happiness measures that can be combined with self-reports. Indeed, biological or physiological indicators, such as specific brain activation patterns (Urry et al., 2004), cortisol and heart rates (Steptoe et al., 2005), immunological parameters (Miller, Chen, & Cole, 2009) and electrophysiological measures (Diener et al., 1997) have shown to be potentially useful in complementing classical self-report happiness measures, as have recordings of facial emotional expressions (Harker & Keltner, 2001). The results of these alternative happiness measures highly converge with those of self-reports.

Differences in Scaling: What Scale Should be Chosen?

In happiness research, it is common to utilize a large variety of rating scales, such as rating scales with 3–11 points or more or face scales, to capture the construct of interest. Because of the use of different scales, it is difficult to make comparisons between happiness results from various investigations. For instance, it is well-known that the use of differing scales can lead to diverging answers (Lim, 2008). What are the critical points in creating response scales? What kind of scale should be chosen from a psychometric point of view?

The first issue concerns whether to use an uneven number of scale levels (containing a midpoint) or an even number of scales levels (forcing participants to take a position). Current research on this topic clearly indicates that the first option is preferred over the second one (Berk, 1979; Nowlis, Kahn, & Dhar, 2002; Weijters, Cabooter, & Schillewaert, 2010), as adding a midpoint to rating scales improves the reliability and validity of the judgments obtained, whereas omitting a midpoint forces participants to randomly choose one of the scale points that is closest to the midpoint (Krosnick & Presser, 2010). Thus, when happiness is measured, an uneven number of scale points is recommended.

The second challenge concerns the choice of the right number of answering options in total. In general, if there are many options available, participants are more likely to find a match between their attitude and one of the given answering options (Krosnick & Fabrigar, 1997). This point of view is supported by the finding that reliability rises with an increasing number of answering options (Diener, Lucas, Schimmack, & Helliwell, 2009). But one needs to be cautious, as using too many options can cause ambiguity and feelings of being overwhelmed, which then can lead to enhanced satisficing (Krosnick & Fabrigar, 1997). According to Miller's research in (1956), which was accompanied by the statement of the "magical number seven, plus or minus two" (p. 81), 5–9 scale points should be perfect. In fact, current research underlines this claim in demonstrating that 5- and 7-point scales resulted in the higher reliability and validity scores than other scales (Krosnick, 1999a; Krosnick & Fabrigar, 1997). Some authors even clearly favour a 7-point scale, since it is commonly used in previous studies, it has high sensitivity and reliability, and people are able to classify their opinion precisely (which is more difficult with more scale levels, such as 9 or 11; Berk, 1979; Finstad, 2010; Menold & Tausch, 2015; Rohrmann, 1978; Weijters et al., 2010; Weng, 2004). In sum, research in this field indicates that a 5- or 7-point rating scale should be applied whenever possible.

Another critical issue in scale construction concerns the use of full labelling versus partial labelling of individual scale points. Concerning this topic, researchers clearly favour the first alternative because, on the one hand, respondents admit to preferring it (Krosnick & Fabrigar, 1997) and, on the other hand, they obtain more reliable and valid results (Krosnick, 1999a, b; Krosnick & Fabrigar, 1997; Pasek & Krosnick, 2010). The primary reason for this finding seems to be that an explanation of each scale point facilitates respondents' understanding (Krosnick, 1999b; Pasek & Krosnick, 2010). Thus, defining the verbal label for every scale point is crucial, and researchers need to take care in selecting appropriate and clear labels that at least cover equally distributed intervals along the whole scale (Krosnick, 1999a, b; Krosnick & Fabrigar, 1997). In this way, researchers can obtain benefits from using fully labelled scales.

Another issue concerns the question whether to add numerical labels to already existing verbal labels. Research on this topic shows that people respond to scales containing the same verbal labels but diverging numerical labels differently (0–10 vs. −5 to +5; Krosnick & Fabrigar, 1997; Schwarz, Knäuper, Hippler, Noelle-Neumann, & Clark, 1991), indicating that respondents use numerical labels "to disambiguate the meaning of scale labels, resulting in different interpretations and, accordingly, different subjective scale anchors" (Schwarz et al., 1991, p. 570). Consequently, answers to the same questions obtained by using comparable verbal scale labels but differing numerical labels are difficult to compare. Furthermore, which results ultimately reflect respondents' true attitude remains unclear. Besides the distortion of answering patterns, another disadvantage of additional numerical labels concerns the increased cognitive burden for respondents (Pasek & Krosnick, 2010), which may lead to faster fatigue and a greater number of errors. In sum, research clearly suggests that numerical labels be omitted from rating scales.

Acquiescence caused by the use of agree-disagree rating scales is a common, well-known effect that also needs to be considered, as it can lead to distorted response patterns (Krosnick, 1999a; Saris, Revilla, Krosnick, & Shaeffer, 2010). Krosnick (1999a) listed possible reasons for this phenomenon, such as people's tendency to act politely rather than oppositely in interpersonal situations or to defer to people of higher status. According to his and many other authors' investigations, the best method to eliminate acquiescence is to avoid agree-disagree rating scales when possible and to offer construct-specific response choices instead (e.g., "completely unhappy"—"completely happy"). Scales comprising such answering options have been shown to provide higher quality responses (Saris et al., 2010).

A final issue concerns graphical scales, such as the face scale, which is regularly used in studies of happiness (according to the WDOH, 32 different face scale measures[5]). Such face scales may particularly bring advantages over classical rating scales, as uneducated respondents can use them (Veenhoven, 1984), especially children who are still illiterate, and as they focus on the respondent's happiness evaluation based on their experiences (Veenhoven, 1984). By contrast, respondents perhaps pay too much attention to their emotions, and thus, face scales are meant to exclusively measure the affective happiness component rather than overall happiness (Veenhoven, 1984). Furthermore, to date, validation studies remain pending. Hence, what such scales actually measure and with what level of quality remain unclear. Thus, researchers should be cautious in applying them, as their effects on respondents remain uncertain.

Overall, on the basis of current research, the following recommendations for scale construction can be given: make use of (i) an uneven number of scale levels (with a midpoint) with at most (ii) 5 or 7 points and (iii) full scale level labelling. In contrast, omit (iv) additional numerical labels and (v) agree-disagree rating scales whenever possible. Be cautious with (vi) graphical scales, such as the face scale, as research on their psychometric quality is still pending.

Differences in Study Construction: Cross-Sectional Versus Longitudinal Design?

According to the WDOH, cross-sectional data on happiness constitutes the vast majority of such data in comparison with longitudinal data (1,599 measures vs. 108 measures[6]). This finding is in line with the feelings of researchers claiming that cross-sectional studies compose the standard in happiness research despite their various shortcomings (Diener, 2012; Diener et al., 1999). Criticized points in particularly are that by exclusively relying on cross-sectional designs, causal directions remain unclear (Diener, 2012; Diener et al., 1999; Graham, 2005), and happiness ratings "can be disproportionately influenced by brief peak moods" (Pressman & Cohen, 2005, p. 963). To solve the latter problem, longitudinal designs can offer an aggregated estimate over the course of several points in time (Diener et al., 2003; Pressman & Cohen, 2005). By doing so, especially measurement errors can be avoided or at least reduced (Graham, 2005). Further advantages of applying a longitudinal design are that it allows a much deeper investigation of the underlying processes (cp. Pressman & Cohen, 2005) and the correction of unobserved personality traits (Graham, 2005).

An exemplary method that can measure "daily moods over an extended period" (Sandvik et al., 1993, p. 321) is the experience sampling method (ESM: Csikszentmihalyi & Larsen, 2014; Csikszentmihalyi, Larson, & Prescott, 1977; Hektner, Schmidt, & Csikszentmihalyi, 2007) also known as ecological momentary assessment (EMA: Stone & Shiffman, 1994; Stone, Shiffman & DeVries, 1999). In investigations applying this method, researchers contact their respondents via a beeper (or nowadays via mobile devices; MacKerron, 2012) several times a day over the course of a longer time period and ask them to complete questions on what they currently do,

[5] As assessed on January 31st, 2017.

[6] As assessed on January 31st, 2017.

where, with whom, and how they feel meanwhile. A recent study indicates that using their smartphone, respondents needed only 30 s to accomplish a single notification (Hendriks, Ludwigs, & Veenhoven, 2016). In this way, the ESM/EMA constitutes a method that can be applied in longitudinal panel designs that aim at surveying respondents in especially short time intervals (multi-moment assessment) in order to obtain additional time-use information. Besides the abovementioned benefits of a longitudinal design, the ESM/EMA offer more valid results than those obtained in cross-sectional studies with retrospective happiness assessments because memory on happiness should be more precise for a relatively brief time period than for a longer time period that needs to be retrieved (Sandvik et al., 1993). In addition, respondents may be more honest because admitting that a particular day was bad, as doing so is not as grave as claiming that their whole life is a mess (Sandvik et al., 1993). The ESM/EMA is additionally beneficial for assessing happiness in people who have problems with their memory because they can no longer possess based on their hippocampus. Such people exclusively live in the present and are thus still able to judge their current feelings (cp. Diener et al., 1997).

In sum, the still often used cross-sectional designs need to be extended by more sophisticated longitudinal designs (Diener, 2012; Diener et al., 1999; Frey & Stutzer, 2002; Graham, 2005). Such use of longitudinal designs seems to be especially urgent since recent investigations applying longitudinal designs have revealed deviating results from those obtained by regular cross-sectional design usage (Diener, 2012). As an example, the ESM/EMA offers a beneficial multi-moment assessment method to capture happiness in the long term.

To complete this psychometric section, Table 1.4 summarizes all recommendations for high quality happiness measure construction, derived from the previous elaborated literature review and discussion. The next section addresses the numerous challenges that can arise when the highest psychometric standard is implemented in real investigations.

Measure Applicability

Researchers who decide to incorporate happiness measures in their investigations generally use measures with the highest quality. Nevertheless, specific research questions, contexts or populations of interest may cause researchers to think about alternative, more feasible measures. The following section discusses circumstances that can justify the use of happiness measures that do not fulfil highest criteria for psychometric quality. Nevertheless, possible approaches that may help researchers revise the truthfulness of one's own reasons for not attaching to the highest psychometric standards are also presented.

Differences in Time Frames

Above we showed that from a psychometric viewpoint, there is currently no reason to avoid using a specific time frame when constructing happiness measures. Consequently, the time frame that the researcher uses strongly depends on the question of interest and the population surveyed. Imagine, for example, an investigation in a company that needs to be conducted to derive significant interventions for the sake of

Table 1.4 Summary of recommendations about how to construct high quality happiness measures, as described in Sect. 3.2 in detail

Topic (referring section)	Recommendation(s)
Time frames	Use the time frame that fits your research question, context and/or population best
Single-item measure versus multiple-item measure	Prefer multiple-item happiness measures over single-item happiness measures
Self-report versus rating by others	Complement self-reports of happiness with further methods with their own strengths, such as ratings by others, biological and physiological indicators or recordings of facial emotional expressions
Scaling	Make use of: (i) an uneven number of scale levels (containing a midpoint) with at most (ii) 5 or 7 points and (iii) full scale level labelling. In contrast, omit (iv) additional numerical labels and (v) agree-disagree rating scales whenever possible. Be cautious with (vi) graphical scales, such as the face scale
Cross-sectional versus longitudinal design	Implement longitudinal designs whenever possible

achieving higher well-being and productivity among employees in the long term. In this case, the status quo is the main interest, and thus, a relatively short time frame is useful. In contrast, a further example illustrates that for another context, a longer time frame could be beneficial. Indeed, national (panel) surveys are often conducted at regular time intervals of about one year or more (such as the Eurobarometer Survey: EC, 2016; Gallup World Poll: Gesis, 2012; Socio-Economic Panel [SOEP]: DIW, 2016; World Values Survey: WVS Association, 2016), and they generally strive to determine the nation's happiness over the course of several years or even decades. Thus, covering the entire time interval from one survey to another is of tremendous relevance, and determining average happiness in the previous year, for example, does make sense such these circumstances. Furthermore, the importance of time frame in creating happiness measures is demonstrated in the following example: Some people no longer have a hippocampus, leading to cognitive impairment for past memories (cp. Diener et al., 1997). Such people are exclusively able to judge their feelings with respect to the present. In addition, children have difficulties in remembering past experiences, owing to maturity (Friedman & Kemp, 1998; Hayne & Imuta, 2011). Consequently, for both target groups, responses of higher validity can be obtained by utilizing relatively short time frames.

Differences in Number of Items: Single-Item Measures Versus Multiple-Item Measures

From a psychometric perspective, we showed above that multiple-item measures are better than single-item measures even though the latter can still be used without losing too much quality. In fact, there may be specific conditions under which the use of single-item measures may be preferable because of practicability issues. For example, large-scale (panel) surveys aim at depicting respondents' views on a huge variety of topics. Consequently, the capacity to evaluate every topic remains limited, meaning that only a few items can be used, as the burden on respondent should be kept at an acceptable level (cp. Diener et al., 2003; Lucas & Donnellan, 2012). Thus, this context may justify the use of lower quality single-item measures instead of multiple-item measures. Another scenario that may lead to the use of single-item measures as a favourable approach arises as soon as observations are required in very short time intervals (such as multi-moment assessments). Then, multiple-item measures might cause tremendously high drop-out rates because respondents associate too much effort with the corresponding investigation. Hence, in this case, single-item measures could be the preferable option. A further critical issue can arise if the survey aims to investigate people with cognitive problems, such as attentional deficits. For this population, it might be beneficial to keep the investigation as brief as possible in order to guarantee the highest validity attainable. Furthermore, imagine a survey target population that currently exercises everyday life and that is to be surveyed spontaneously during, for instance, walking through a pedestrian zone. Such a situation frequently evolves when market research is conducted among the general population. A crucial issue is that people often have numerous responsibilities in the moment and are thus not willing to interrupt them in order to complete a questionnaire of 250 items. Consequently, keeping the survey as short as possible by only using single-item measures for every construct should help obtain reasonable participation rates.

In sum, there are several understandable reasons for not choosing the highest psychometric standard and instead using single-item measures only. But where is the proof that all these assumptions reflect reality? Hence, the validity of these reasons should be considered. In this way, researchers can verify whether response rates actually diminish, whether the perceived burden for respondents actually rises and whether cognitive disabled persons actually provide answers of lower quality. In the best case, all concerns can be proved as unfounded, and thus, there are no longer reasons to further omit multiple-item measures as more valid measures of the happiness construct. One opportunity to verify the abovementioned assumptions consists in simply splitting the sample, where half completes the single-item version and the other half completes the longer, multiple-item version. Another possibility for longitudinal designs, such as multi-moment assessment or classical national-wide panel surveys, can be to generally use the single-item version but to sometimes use the more intense, multiple-item version. With these two suggestions, researchers can revise their reasons for choosing single-item measures and maybe change their view.

Differences in Measurement Techniques: Self-report Versus Ratings by Others?

Above, we noted that from a psychometric view, self-reports do not deliver information of the highest quality possible because of likely answering distortions. Thus, the use of complementary measures is recommended to obtain more valid results. But despite the weaknesses of self-reports, we also stated that self-reports can capture meaningful information on happiness. Thus, depending on context and population, using only self-reports or only ratings by others can be justifiable. As previously mentioned, especially large-scale (panel) surveys need to take care of respondents' burden and thus limit the number of items used to cover the constructs of interest. In addition, monetary aspects play a role, as funding made available for such studies is definite. Overall, both arguments indicate that particularly for large-scale studies, it can be more feasible to use only self-reports for happiness instead of adding further, complementary measures, such as ratings by others. By contrast, for extremely mentally disabled persons, it can make sense to generally omit self-reports and apply alternative measures to assess individuals' level of happiness.

As similarly stated above, all these arguments support comprehensible reasons for avoiding the use of complementary happiness measures. Nevertheless, the extent to which these reasons can be considered well-grounded remains unclear. Consequently, these assumptions need to be verified in terms of their correctness: Is the respondent burden actually increased if complementary happiness measures are added to the survey? Is money definitely too restricted as to allow the application of additional measures? Are mentally disabled persons really not able to provide meaningful information about their current happiness? The above suggested methods may help to shed light on these questions.

Differences in Scaling: What Scale Should be Chosen?

It was generally noted that using variously constructed scales can lead to differences in respondents' answers. Thus, if possible, researchers should follow the above recommendations to fulfil the highest psychometric standards. However, there are exceptional situations in which relying on commonly used but lesser quality measures can be beneficial. Some surveys have been conducted for many years and thus have a tradition that cannot be denied. Particularly with respect to comparability issues, keeping the current scaling constant may be a better alternative. Consequently, spontaneously changing the scales used can even cause disadvantages, such as worse comparability with previous investigations. Concerning graphical scales, such as the face scale, it has been claimed that psychometric research in this field is not available yet. Nevertheless, for assessing children and mentally disabled persons, such scales may be the best option. Namely, using alternative rating scales may result in answers of much lower quality, as the respondents are not capable of answering such questions. Thus, using a face scale under such circumstances can definitely make sense. To conclude, it nevertheless needs to be posited that under the premises of a normal population and a completely new survey, researchers should consider the recommendations here concerning scale construction. In this way, the highest quality standards can be achieved.

Differences in Study Construction: Cross-Sectional Versus Longitudinal Design?

From a psychometric point of view, longitudinal designs offer many advantages over cross-sectional designs and should be implemented, if possible. But the context and investigated population are also important, and they can shift the preference towards a cross-sectional design. Imagine, for example, a representative, longitudinal survey conducted among refugees. Such a target group is tremendously difficult to investigate over a longer time period, as many refugees change their living place frequently. Consequently, they may not be able to participate in subsequent surveys and may thus drop out of the panel. Thus, for the group of refugees, a detailed, cross-sectional investigation instead of a longitudinal survey, which has considerable potential to suffer from a high drop-out rate, may be beneficial. However, in the long-term, solutions should be found to facilitate longitudinal investigations on such challenging populations. As will be shown in the following paragraph, applying newly developed, digital technologies implement complex longitudinal designs may be a promising strategy for future studies.

Another critical point in applying longitudinal designs consists in their often extraordinarily high (time and monetary) costs for both respondents and researchers. Consider, for example, the ESM/EMA that was introduced above to depict multi-moment assessment, a specific method used in longitudinal designs. When this method is implemented, respondents are asked to complete questions on their happiness, several times a day over the course of a longer time period. In the original study, answers were recorded via paper-pencil usage; thus, respondents needed to carry this equipment with them all the time (Csikszentmihalyi et al., 1977). Consequently, researchers are required to make ESM sheets and pencils available, and in the end, they need to manually transfer the entire data sets to the PC. Overall, it is not surprising that the ESM/EMA is repeatedly described as a rather time consuming and costly method to capture happiness during everyday life (Dolan & White, 2007; Kahneman, Krueger, Schkade, Schwarz, & Stone, 2004b; Krueger & Schkade, 2008). It was also criticized that the ESM/EMA is able to show only excerpts of everyday life instead of depicting the whole day and thus allowing precise time use information (Kahneman et al., 2004b). Because of these shortcomings, Kahneman and colleagues (2004a, b) developed the *Day Reconstruction Method* (DRM), where respondents are regularly asked to reconstruct their prior day in single episodes, for instance, by filling in a diary (e.g., 8–9 o'clock breakfast, 9–12 o'clock work). Thus, they indicate which activities they undertook in which time period, where they did, with whom, and how happy they were doing so. In addition, the DRM was initially primarily implemented via paper-pencil format (Kahneman et al., 2004b). Although it could be found that DRM data highly converges with ESM/EMA data (Kahneman & Krueger, 2006; Kahneman et al., 2004b), it is not necessary to abandon the ESM/EMA completely. On the contrary, this method especially needs to become more efficient for researchers to apply and for respondents to use. However, the DRM would also benefit from such an approach. As mentioned before, most DRMs are still recorded via paper and pencil. For this purpose, the current digitalization process brings new possibilities for applying both methods in a more efficient way than before.

In recent times, diverse researchers launched mobile phone applications containing ESM/EMA (Killingsworth & Gilbert, 2010[7]; MacKerron, 2011[8]) and additionally DRM (Hendriks et al. 2016). In this way, the study of Hendriks et al. (2016), for example, shows the enormous cost and time efficiency obtained by conducting the study on a digital basis: Over the course of two weeks, more than 16,000 happiness ratings and 4000 diaries could be achieved with only a single researcher running the whole study and total costs of about 500€ (excluded are costs of the researcher). The burden for every respondent in terms of time was about 2 h a week at maximum, and all data were automatically saved and analysed via app without the need to manually code and evaluate the data. In sum, it becomes obvious what opportunities can arise when researchers dare to embrace new digital technologies in forthcoming investigations. Thus, it is promising that newly invented technologies can facilitate the implementation of longitudinal and especially multi-moment assessment designs.

1.3 Summary and Prospects

At the beginning of this book chapter, we showed that it is worthwhile to research happiness since it brings a large variety of benefits for every individual and for society. Concurrently, we need to find out more about this construct to achieve the ambitious goal of making people happier in general. In particular, appropriate measures are needed to capture the happiness of various people in different situations as validly as possible. Based on the WDOH, the status quo of existing happiness measures was noted, with a particular focus on their strengths and weaknesses. Researchers should consider these findings in selecting their happiness measures in future investigations. Particularly the continuing digitalization process will enable happiness researchers to easier include multi-moment and multi-method assessments in their studies. If they do so, results will be obtained that were impossible to obtain a few years ago. However, considerable progress needs to be made in this field with respect to the following questions: How can we guarantee representative samples especially with respect to extremely young and elder respondents? Do respondents change their behaviour over the course of the investigation, owing to repeated monitoring (cp. Dolan & White, 2007)? There are also certainly many other questions one can think of. Answering these questions to guarantee high quality measures by using new technologies should be an important goal of forthcoming studies.

To conclude, we can state that despite initial concerns about the question whether happiness could be measured satisfactorily, we can now state that considerable progress has been made in this field. However, researchers should be cautious about keeping up to date with the newest findings on the psychometrics of the happiness measures. If they discover weaknesses in their measures and if it is feasible to revise them, they should dare to do so to guarantee the highest quality standards.

---

[7]Free app download: http://www.trackyourhappiness.com (lastly retrieved on January 31st, 2017).
[8]Free app download: http://www.mappiness.org.uk (lastly retrieved on January 31st, 2017).

In particular, openness towards new developments owing to digitalization processes is required, as arising methods in this field are promising for further enhancing currently available happiness measures.

References

Aknin, L. B., Sandstrom, G. M., Dunn, E. W., & Norton, M. I. (2011). Investing in others: Prosocial spending for (pro) social change. In R. Biswas-Diener (Ed.), *Positive psychology as social change* (pp. 219–234). Netherlands: Springer.

Allianz Deutschland AG & RWI (Rheinisch-Westfälisches Institut für Wirtschaftsforschung e.V.). (2011). Depression – Wie die Krank- heit unsere Seele belastet. Munich, Germany: Lohse Druckgesellschaft. Retrieved February 17, 2016, from http://www.rwi-essen.de/media/content/pages/publikationen/sonstige/Allianz-Report-Depression.pdf.

Andrews, F. M., & Withey, S. B. (1976). *Social indicators of well-being: Americans' perceptions of life quality*. New York, USA: Plenum Press.

Bacon, N., Brophy, M., Mguni, N., Mulgan, G., & Shandro, A. (2010). *The state of happiness: Can public policy shape peoples wellbeing and resilience?* London, UK: The Young Foundation.

Berk, R. A. (1979). The construction of rating instruments for faculty evaluation: A review of methodological issues. *The Journal of Higher Education, 50*(5), 650–669.

Bjørnskov, C. (2010). How comparable are the Gallup World Poll life satisfaction data? *Journal of Happiness Studies, 11*(1), 41–60.

Bradburn, N. M. (1969). *The structure of psychological well-being*. Chicago, USA: Aldine Publishing.

Bradburn, N. M., & Caplovitz, D. (1965). *Reports on happiness: A pilot study of behavior related to mental health*. Chicago, USA: Aldine Publishing.

Bruni, L. (2010). The happiness of sociality. Economics and eudaimonia: A necessary encounter. *Rationality and Society, 22*(4), 383–406.

Busseri, M. A., & Sadava, S. W. (2011). A review of the tripartite structure of subjective well-being: Implications for conceptualization, operationalization, analysis, and synthesis. *Personality and Social Psychology Review, 5*(3), 290–314.

Buttel, F. H., & Martinson, O. B. (1977). Ideology and social indicators of the quality of life. *Social Indicators Research, 4*(1), 353–369.

Cameron, D. (2006, July 20). *General well-being speech*. Retrieved February 17, 2016, from https://toryspeeches.files.wordpress.com/2013/11/david-cameron-general-well-being-speech.pdf.

Clark, E., & Senik, C. (2011). Is happiness different from flourishing? Cross-country evidence from the ESS. *Revue d'économie poli-tique, 121*(1), 17–34.

Clark, A., Georgellis, Y., & Sanfey, P. (1998). Job satisfaction, wage changes and quits: Evidence from Germany. *Research in Labor Economics, 17,* 95–121.

Commission of the European Communities. (2009). GDP and beyond: Measuring progress in a changing world. Communication from the Commission to the Council and the European Parliament. Retrieved February 17, 2016, from http://eur-lex.europa.eu/legal-content/EN/TXT/PDF/?uri=CELEX:52009DC0433&from=EN.

Constantinople, A. (1967). Perceived instrumentality of the college as a measure of attitudes toward college. *Journal of Personality and Social Psychology, 5*(2), 196–201.

Cropanzano, R., & Wright, T. A. (1999). A 5-year study of change in the relationship between well-being and job performance. *Consulting Psychology Journal: Practice and Research, 51*(4), 252–265.

Csikszentmihalyi, M., & Larson, R. (2014). Validity and reliability of the experience-sampling method. In M. Csikszentmihalyi (Ed.), *Flow and the foundations of positive psychology* (Chapter 3, pp. 35–54). Dordrecht, The Netherlands: Springer.

Csikszentmihalyi, M., Larson, R., & Prescott, S. (1977). The ecology of adolescent activity and experience. *Journal of Youth and Adolescence, 6*(3), 281–294.
Cunningham, M. R., Steinberg, J., & Grev, R. (1980). Wanting to and having to help: Separate motivations for positive mood and guilt-induced helping. *Journal of Personality and Social Psychology, 38*(2), 181–192.
Danner, D. D., Snowdon, D. A., & Friesen, W. V. (2001). Positive emotions in early life and longevity: Findings from the nun study. *Journal of Personality and Social Psychology, 80*(5), 804–813.
DGPPN (Deutsche Gesellschaft für Psychiatrie und Psychotherapie, Psychosomatik und Nervenheilkunde). (2013). Gemeinsam für psychische Gesundheit: Erwartungen der DGPPN an die Gesundheitspolitik (Brochure). Retrieved February 17, 2016, from https://www.dgppn.de/fileadmin/user_upload/_medien/download/pdf/Broschüren/DGP_Broschuere_Politik_2013_gesamt-Einzelseiten.pdf.
Di Tella, R., & MacCulloch, R. (2008). Gross national happiness as an answer to the Easterlin Paradox? *Journal of Development Economics, 86*(1), 22–42.
Diener, E. (2000). Subjective well-being: The science of happiness and a proposal for a national index. *American Psychologist, 55*(1), 34–43.
Diener, E. (2012). New findings and future directions for subjective well-being research. *American Psychologist, 67*(8), 590–597.
Diener, E., & Chan, M. Y. (2011). Happy people live longer: Subjective well-being contributes to health and longevity. *Applied Psychology: Health and Well-Being, 3*(1), 1–43.
Diener, E., & Larsen, R. J. (1984). Temporal stability and cross situational consistency of affective, behavioral, and cognitive responses. *Journal of Personality and Social Psychology, 47*(4), 580–592.
Diener, E., & Seligman, M. E. (2004). Beyond money toward an economy of well-being. *Psychological Science in the Public Interest, 5*(1), 1–31.
Diener, E., Lucas, R. E., & Scollon, C. N. (2006). Beyond the hedonic treadmill: Revising the adaptation theory of well-being. *American Psychologist, 61*(4), 305–314.
Diener, E., Sandvik, E., Pavot, W., & Gallagher, D. (1991). Response artifacts in the measurement of subjective well-being. *Social Indicators Research, 24*(1), 35–56.
Diener, E., Scollon, C. N., & Lucas, R. E. (2003). The evolving concept of subjective well-being: The multifaceted nature of happiness. *Advances in Cell Aging and Gerontology, 15,* 187–219.
Diener, E., Suh, E., & Oishi, S. (1997). Recent findings on subjective well-being. *Indian Journal of Clinical Psychology, 24,* 25–41.
Diener, E., Suh, E., Lucas, R. E., & Smith, H. L. (1999). Subjective well-being: Three decades of progress. *Psychological Bulletin, 125*(2), 276–302.
Diener, E., Lucas, R. E., Oishi, S., & Suh, E. M. (2002a). Looking up and looking down: Weighting good and bad information in life satisfaction judgments. *Personality and Social Psychology Bulletin, 28*(4), 437–445.
Diener, E., Nickerson, C., Lucas, R. E., & Sandvik, E. (2002b). Dispositional affect and job outcomes. *Social Indicators Research, 59*(3), 229–259.
Diener, E., Lucas, R. E., Schimmack, U., & Helliwell, J. F. (2009). *Well-being for public policy.* Oxford, England: University Press.
Diener, E., Wirtz, D., Tov, W., Kim-Prieto, C., Choi, D. W., Oishi, S., et al. (2010). New well-being measures: Short scales to assess flourishing and positive and negative feelings. *Social Indicators Research, 97*(2), 143–156.
DIW (German Institute for Economic Research). (2016). *Socio-economic panel* (website). Retrieved March 22, 2016, from http://www.diw.de/en/soep.
Dolan, P., & White, M. P. (2007). How can measures of subjective well-being be used to inform public policy? *Perspectives on Psychological Science, 2*(1), 71–85.
Dolan, P., Peasgood, T., & White, M. (2006). *Review of research on the influences on personal well-being and application to policy making*. London, England: DEFRA.

Dolan, P., Peasgood, T., & White, M. (2008). Do we really know what makes us happy? A review of the economic literature on the factors associated with subjective well-being. *Journal of Economic Psychology, 29*(1), 94–122.
Easterlin, R. A. (2003). Explaining happiness. *Proceedings of the National Academy of Sciences, 100*(19), 11176–11183.
EC (European Commission). (2016). *Eurobarometer surveys* (website). Retrieved March 22, 2016, from http://ec.europa.eu/public_opinion/index_en.htm.
Ehrhardt, J. J., Saris, W. E., & Veenhoven, R. (2000). Stability of life-satisfaction over time. *Journal of Happiness Studies, 1*(2), 177–205.
Eid, M., & Diener, E. (1999). Intraindividual variability in affect: Reliability, validity, and personality correlates. *Journal of Personality and Social Psychology, 76*(4), 662–676.
Else-Quest, N. M., Hyde, J. S., & DeLamater, J. D. (2005). Context counts: Long-term sequelae of premarital intercourse or abstinence. *Journal of Sex Research, 42*(2), 102–112.
Fernández-Dols, J. M., & Ruiz-Belda, M. A. (1995). Are smiles a sign of happiness? Gold medal winners at the Olympic games. *Journal of Personality and Social Psychology, 69*(6), 1113–1119.
Finstad, K. (2010). Response interpolation and scale sensitivity: Evidence against 5-point scales. *Journal of Usability Studies, 5*(3), 104–110.
Flügel, J. C. (1925). A quantitative study of feeling and emotion in everyday life. *British Journal of Psychology. General Section, 15*(4), 318–355.
Fordyce, M. W. (1977). Development of a program to increase personal happiness. *Journal of Counseling Psychology, 24*(6), 511–521.
Frey, B. S., & Stutzer, A. (2002). What can economists learn from happiness research? *Journal of Economic Literature, 40*(2), 402–435.
Friedman, W. J., & Kemp, S. (1998). The effects of elapsed time and retrieval on young children's judgments of the temporal distances of past events. *Cognitive Development, 13*(3), 335–367.
Frijters, P. (2000). Do individuals try to maximize general satisfaction? *Journal of Economic Psychology, 21*(3), 281–304.
Fujita, F., & Diener, E. (2005). Life satisfaction set point: Stability and change. *Journal of Personality and Social Psychology, 88*(1), 158–164.
George, J. M. (1991). State or trait: Effects of positive mood on prosocial behaviors at work. *Journal of Applied Psychology, 76*(2), 299–307.
Gesis. (2012). Zum Gallup World Poll. Abgerufen unter: http://www.gesis.org/fileadmin/upload/dienstleistung/veranstaltungen_fortbildungen/workshops/Infotext_GALLUP_WS_040912.pdf. Retrieved from March 22, 2016.
Goldings, H. J. (1954). On the avowal and projection of happiness. *Journal of Personality, 23*(1), 30–47.
Graham, C. (2005). The economics of happiness—Insights on globalization from a novel approach. *World Economics, 6*(3), 41–55.
Haas, O., & Janssen, B. (2012). *Happiness steckt an. Personalwirtschaft, 42*(8), 56–57.
Harker, L., & Keltner, D. (2001). Expressions of positive emotions in women's college yearbook pictures and their relationship to personality and life outcomes across adulthood. *Journal of Personality and Social Psychology, 80*(1), 112–124.
Harter, J. K., Schmidt, F. L., Asplund, J., & Kilham, E. A. (2010). Causal impact of employee work perceptions on the bottom line of organizations. *Perspectives on Psychological Science, 5*, 378–389.
Hayne, H., & Imuta, K. (2011). Episodic memory in 3-and 4-year-old children. *Developmental Psychobiology, 53*(3), 317–322.
Hektner, J. M., Schmidt, J. A., & Csikszentmihalyi, M. (2007). Psychometrics of ESM data. In J. M. Hektner, J. A. Schmidt, & M. Csikszentmihalyi (Eds.), *Experience sampling method: Measuring the quality of everyday life* (Chapter 6, pp. 103–122). Thousand Oaks, USA: Sage.
Hendriks, M., Ludwigs, K., & Veenhoven, R. (2016). Why are locals happier than internal migrants? The role of daily life. *Social Indicators Research, 125*(2), 481–508.

Holder, M. D., Coleman, B., & Wallace, J. M. (2010). Spirituality, religiousness, and happiness in children aged 8–12 years. *Journal of Happiness Studies, 11,* 131–150.

Huppert, F. A., Marks, N., Clark, A., Siegrist, J., Stutzer, A., Vittersø, J., et al. (2009). Measuring well-being across Europe: Description of the ESS well-being module and preliminary findings. *Social Indicators Research, 91*(3), 301–315.

Isen, A. M. (1970). Success, failure, attention, and reaction to others: The warm glow of success. *Journal of Personality and Social Psychology, 15*(4), 294–301.

Isen, A. M., Daubman, K. A., & Nowicki, G. P. (1987). Positive affect facilitates creative problem solving. *Journal of Personality and Social Psychology, 52*(6), 1122–1131.

Jolly, D. (2009, September 14). GDP seen as inadequate measure of economic health. *The New York Times*, p. 14. Retrieved February 17, 2016, from http://www.nytimes.com/2009/09/15/business/global/15gdp.html?_r=0.

Journal of Happiness Studies. (2016). Dordrecht, The Netherlands: Springer. Retrieved February18, 2016, from http://link.springer.com/journal/10902.

Judge, T. A., & Kammeyer-Mueller, J. D. (2011). Happiness as a societal value. *The Academy of Management Perspectives, 25*(1), 30–41.

Judge, T. A., & Watanabe, S. (1993). Another look at the job satisfaction-life satisfaction relationship. *Journal of Applied Psychology, 78*(6), 939–948.

Judge, T. A., Thoresen, C. J., Bono, J. E., & Patton, G. K. (2001). The job satisfaction-job performance relationship: A qualitative and quantitative review. *Psychological Bulletin, 127*(3), 376–407.

Kahneman, D. (1994). New challenges to the rationality assumption. *Journal of Institutional and Theoretical Economics, 150*(1), 18–36.

Kahneman, D., & Krueger, A. B. (2006). Developments in the measurement of subjective well-being. *The Journal of Economic Perspectives, 20*(1), 3–24.

Kahneman, D., Krueger, A. B., Schkade, D., Schwarz, N., & Stone, A. (2004a). Toward national well-being accounts. *American Economic Review, 94*(2), 429–434.

Kahneman, D., Krueger, A. B., Schkade, D. A., Schwarz, N., & Stone, A. A. (2004b). A survey method for characterizing daily life experience: The day reconstruction method. *Science, 306,* 1776–1780.

Kammann, R., & Flett, R. (1983). *Sourcebook for measuring well-being with Affectometer 2.* Dunedin, New Zealand: Why Not? Foundation.

Kantor, H. I., Milton, L. J., & Ernst, M. L. (1978). Comparative psychologic effects of estrogen administration on institutional and noninstitutional elderly women. *Journal of the American Geriatrics Society, 26*(1), 9–16.

Killingsworth, M. A., & Gilbert, D. T. (2010). A wandering mind is an unhappy mind. *Science, 330*(6006), 932.

Koivumaa-Honkanen, H., Honkanen, R., Koskenvuo, M., & Kaprio, J. (2003). Self-reported happiness in life and suicide in ensuing 20 years. *Social Psychiatry and Psychiatric Epidemiology, 38*(5), 244–248.

Krosnick, J. A. (1999a). Maximizing questionnaire quality. In J. P. Robinson, P. R. Shaver, L. S. Wrightsman, J. P. Robinson, P. R. Shaver, & L. S. Wrightsman (Eds.), *Measures of political attitudes* (Chapter 2, pp. 37–57). San Diego, USA: Academic Press.

Krosnick, J. A. (1999b). Survey research. *Annual Review of Psychology, 50,* 537–567.

Krosnick, J. A., & Fabrigar, L. R. (1997). Designing rating scales for effective measurement in surveys. In L. Lyberg, P. Biemer, M. Collins, E. de Leeuw, C. Dippo, N. Schwarz, & D. Trewin (Eds.), *Survey measurement and process quality* (Chapter 6, pp. 141–164). New York, USA: Wiley.

Krosnick, J. A., & Presser, S. (2010). Question and questionnaire design. *Handbook of Survey Research, 2,* 263–314.

Krueger, A. B., & Schkade, D. A. (2008). The reliability of subjective well-being measures. *Journal of Public Economics, 92*(8), 1833–1845.

Larsen, R. J., Diener, E. D., & Emmons, R. A. (1985). An evaluation of subjective well-being measures. *Social Indicators Research, 17*(1), 1–17.

Layard, R. (2005). *Happiness: Lessons from a new science*. New York, NY: Penguin Press.

Lemon, B. W., Bengtson, V. L., & Peterson, J. A. (1972). An exploration of the activity theory of aging: Activity types and life satisfaction among in-movers to a retirement community. *Journal of Gerontology, 27*(4), 511–523.

Lepper, H. S. (1998). Use of other-reports to validate subjective well-being measures. *Social Indicators Research, 44*(3), 367–379.

Levy, S., & Guttman, L. (1975). Structure and dynamics of worries. *Sociometry, 38*(4), 445–473.

Lim, H.-E. (2008). The use of different happiness rating scales: Bias and comparison problem? *Social Indicators Research, 87*(2), 259–267.

Lu, L. (2001). Understanding happiness: A look into the Chinese folk psychology. *Journal of Happiness Studies, 2*, 407–432.

Lucas, R. E., & Donnellan, M. B. (2012). Estimating the reliability of single-item life satisfaction measures: Results from four national panel studies. *Social Indicators Research, 105*(3), 323–331.

Lucas, R. E., Diener, E., & Suh, E. (1996). Discriminant validity of well-being measures. *Journal of Personality and Social Psychology, 71*(3), 616–628.

Lyubomirsky, S., King, L., & Diener, E. (2005). The benefits of frequent positive affect: Does happiness lead to success? *Psychological Bulletin, 131*(6), 803–855.

MacKerron, G. (2011). *Happiness and environmental quality*. Dissertation, The London School of Economics and Political Science, Great Britain. Retrieved March 22, 2016, from https://core.ac.uk/download/files/170/6590187.pdf.

MacKerron, G. (2012). Happiness Economics from 35 000 feet. *Journal of Economic Surveys, 26*(4), 705–735.

Mathers, C. D., & Loncar, D. (2006). Projections of global mortality and burden of disease from 2002 to 2030. *PLoS Medicine, 3*(11), 2011–2030.

Menold, N., & Tausch, A. (2015). Measurement of latent variables with different rating scales testing reliability and measurement equivalence by varying the verbalization and number of categories. *Sociological Methods & Research*, 1–22.

Michalos, A. C. (1980). Satisfaction and happiness. *Social Indicators Research, 8*(4), 385–422.

Michalos, A. C., & Kahlke, P. M. (2010). Stability and sensitivity in perceived quality of life measures: Some panel results. *Social Indicators Research, 98*(3), 403–434.

Miller, G. A. (1956). The magical number seven, plus or minus two: Some limits on our capacity for processing information. *Psychological Review, 63*(2), 81–97.

Miller, G. E., Chen, E., & Cole, S. W. (2009). Healh psychology: Developing biologically plausible models linking the social world and physical health. *Annual Review of Psychology, 60*, 501–524.

Nowlis, S. M., Kahn, B. E., & Dhar, R. (2002). Coping with ambivalence: The effect of removing a neutral option on consumer attitude and preference judgments. *Journal of Consumer Research, 29*(3), 319–334.

Nussbaum, M. C. (2005). Mill between Aristotle and Bentham. In L. Bruni & P. L. Porta (Eds.), *Economics and happiness: Framing the analysis* (1st ed., Chapter 6, pp. 170–183). Oxford, England: University Press.

OECD (Organisation for Economic Co-operation and Development). (2013). *OECD Guidelines on measuring subjective well-being*. Paris, France: Author. Retrieved February 18, 2016, from http://dx.doi.org/10.1787/9789264191655-en.

Office for National Statistics. (2012). *First ONS annual experimental subjective well-being results*. Retrieved February 26, 2016, from http://www.ons.gov.uk.

Oishi, S. (2012). *The psychological wealth of nations: Do happy people make a happy society?* Malden, MA: Wiley-Blackwell.

Oswald, A. J., Proto, E., & Sgroi, D. (2009). *Happiness and productivity*. IZA Discussion Paper No. 4645. Retrieved February 17, 2016, from http://hdl.handle.net/10419/35451.

Pasek, J., & Krosnick, J. A. (2010). Optimizing survey questionnaire design in political science: Insights from psychology. In T. C. Davenport, A. S. Gerber, & D. P. Green (Eds.), *The Oxford handbook of American elections and political behavior* (Chapter 3, pp. 27–50). Oxford, England: University Press.

Pavot, W., & Diener, E. (1993). Review of the satisfaction with life scale. *Psychological Assessment, 5*(2), 164–172.

Pfaff, T. (2011). Das Bruttonationalglück aus ordnungspolitischer Sicht: Eine Analyse des Wirtschafts- und Gesellschaftssystems von Bhutan (Working Paper Series des Rates für Sozial- und Wirtschaftsdaten, No. 182). Retrieved February 17, 2016, from http://hdl.handle.net/10419/75326.

Pressman, S. D., & Cohen, S. (2005). Does positive affect influence health? *Psychological Bulletin, 131*(6), 925–971.

Priesner, S. (1999). *Gross national happiness—Bhutan's vision of development and its challenges*. Discussion Paper. Retrieved February 17, 2016, from http://crossasia-repository.ub.uni-heidelberg.de/320/1/GNH_Ch3_Priesner.pdf.

Priller, E., & Schupp, J. (2011). Social and economic characteristics of financial and blood donors in Germany. *DIW Economic Bulletin, 1*(6), 23–30.

Rässler, S., & Riphahn, R. T. (2006). Survey item nonresponse and its treatment. *Allgemeines Statistisches Archiv, 90,* 217–232.

Rohrmann, B. (1978). Empirische Studien zur Entwicklung von Antwortskalen für die sozialwissenschaftliche Forschung. *Zeitschrift für Sozialpsychologie, 9*(3), 222–245.

Ryan, R. M., & Deci, E. L. (2000). Self-determination theory and the facilitation of intrinsic motivation, social development, and well-being. *American Psychologist, 55*(1), 68–78.

Ryan, R. M., & Deci, E. L. (2001). On happiness and human potentials: A review of research on hedonic and eudaimonic well-being. *Annual Review of Psychology, 52*(1), 141–166.

Sacks, D. W., Stevenson, B., & Wolfers, J. (2010). *Subjective well-being, income, economic development and growth.* Working Paper No. w16441. Retrieved February 29, 2016, from http://www.nber.org/papers/w16441.

Sandvik, E., Diener, E., & Seidlitz, L. (1993). Subjective well-being: The convergence and stability of self-report and non-self-report measures. *Journal of Personality, 61*(3), 317–342.

Saris, W. E., Revilla, M., Krosnick, J. A., & Shaeffer, E. M. (2010). Comparing questions with Agree/Disagree response options to questions with item-specific response options. *Survey Research Methods, 4,* 61–79.

Schneider, L., & Schimmack, U. (2009). Self-informant agreement in well-being ratings: A meta-analysis. *Social Indicators Research, 94*(3), 363–376.

Schwarz, N. (1988). Stimmung als Information: Zum Einfluß von Stimmungen und Emotionen auf evaluative Urteile. *Psychologische Rundschau, 39,* 148–159.

Schwarz, N., & Clore, G. L. (1983). Mood, misattribution, and judgments of well-being: Informative and directive functions of affective states. *Journal of Personality and Social Psychology, 45*(3), 513–523.

Schwarz, N., & Strack, N. (1991). Evaluating one's life: A judgement model of subjective well-being. In F. Strack, M. Argyle, & N. Schwarz (Eds.), *Subjective well-being: An interdisciplinary perspective* (1st ed., Chapter 3, pp. 27–48). Oxford, England: Pergamon Press.

Schwarz, N., & Strack, F. (1999). Reports of subjective well-being: Judgmental processes and their methodological implications. In D. Kahneman, E. Diener, & N. Schwarz (Eds.), *Well-being: The foundations of hedonic psychology* (Chapter 4, pp. 61–84). New York, USA: Russell Sage Foundation.

Schwarz, N., Strack, F., Kommer, D., & Wagner, D. (1987). Soccer, rooms, and the quality of your life: Mood effects on judgments of satisfaction with life in general and with specific domains. *European Journal of Social Psychology, 17*(1), 69–79.

Schwarz, N., Knäuper, B., Hippler, H., Noelle-Neumann, E., & Clark, L. (1991). Rating scales: Numeric values may change the meaning of scale labels. *Public Opinion Quarterly, 55,* 570–582.

Seligman, M. E. P., & Csikszentmihalyi, M. (2000). Positive psychology: An introduction. *American Psychologist, 55*(1), 5–14.

Simon, R. W., & Nath, L. E. (2004). Gender and emotion in the United States: Do men and women differ in self-reports of feelings and expressive behavior? *American Journal of Sociology, 109*(5), 1137–1176.

Smith, T. W. (1979). Happiness: Time trends, seasonal variations, intersurvey differences, and other mysteries. *Social Psychology Quarterly, 42*(1), 18–30.

Steptoe, A., Wardle, J., & Marmot, M. (2005). Positive affect and health-related neuroendocrine, cardiovascular, and inflammatory processes. *Proceedings of the National Academy of Sciences of the United States of America, 102*(18), 6508–6512.

Stiglitz, J., Sen, A., & Fitoussi, J. P. (2009). *The measurement of economic performance and social progress revisited. Reflections and overview*. Working paper, No. 2009-33. Retrieved February 17, 2016, from https://hal-sciencespo.archives-ouvertes.fr/file/index/docid/1069384/filename/wp2009-33.pdf.

Stone, A. A., & Shiffman, S. (1994). Ecological momentary assessment (EMA) in behavioral medicine. *Annals of Behavioral Medicine, 16*(3), 199–202.

Stone, A. A., Shiffman, S. S., & DeVries, M. W. (1999). Ecological momentary assessment. In D. Kahneman, E. Diener, & N. Schwarz (Eds.), *Well-being: The foundations of hedonic psychology* (pp. 26–39). New York, USA: Russell Sage Foundation.

Stratton, A. (2010, November 14). Happiness index to gauge Britain's national mood. *The Guardian*, p.14. Retrieved February 17, 2016, from http://www.theguardian.com/lifeandstyle/2010/nov/14/happiness-index-britain-national-mood.

Suh, E., Diener, E., Oishi, S., & Triandis, H. C. (1998). The shifting basis of life satisfaction judgments across cultures: Emotions versus norms. *Journal of Personality and Social Psychology, 74*(2), 482–493.

Sumner, L. W. (1996). *Welfare, happiness and ethics*. New York, USA: Oxford University Press.

Tatarkiewicz, W. (1966). Happiness and time. *Philosophy and Phenomenological Research, 27*(1), 1–10.

The American Declaration of Independence. (1776). Retrieved February 18, 2016, from http://www.ushistory.org/declaration/document/index.html.

Thoits, P. A., & Hewitt, L. N. (2001). Volunteer work and well-being. *Journal of Health and Social Behavior, 42*(2), 115–131.

Urry, H. L., Nitschke, J. B., Dolski, I., Jackson, D. C., Dalton, K. M., Mueller, C. J., ... Davidson, R. J. (2004). Making a life worth living neural correlates of well-being. *Psychological Science, 15*(6), 367–372.

Van Praag, B. M., Frijters, P., & Ferrer-i-Carbonell, A. (2003). The anatomy of subjective well-being. *Journal of Economic Behavior and Organization, 51*(1), 29–49.

Veenhoven, R. (1984). *Conditions of happiness*. Doctoral dissertation. Retrieved February 22, 2016, from http://www2.eur.nl/fsw/research/veenhoven/Pub1980s/84a-full.pdf.

Veenhoven, R. (1991). Questions on happiness: Classical topics, modern answers, blind spots. In F. Strack, M. Argyle, & N. Schwarz (Eds.), *Subjective well-being: An interdisciplinary perspective* (1st ed., Chapter 2, pp. 7–26). Oxford, England: Pergamon Press.

Veenhoven, R. (1994). Is happiness a trait? *Social Indicators Research, 32*(2), 101–160.

Veenhoven, R. (1997). Advances in understanding happiness (English translation). *Revue Québécoise de Psychologie, 18*, 29–74.

Veenhoven, R. (2000). The four qualities of life—Ordering concepts and measures of the good life. *Journal of Happiness Studies, 1*, 1–39.

Veenhoven, R. (2008). Comparability of happiness across nations. *School of Sociology and Social Work Journal, 104*, 211–234.

Veenhoven, R. (2010). Greater happiness for a greater number. Is that possible and desirable? *Journal of Happiness Studies, 11*, 605–629.

Veenhoven, R. (2015). *Classification of happiness measures (world database of happiness, measures of happiness, introductory text)*. Retrieved February 26, 2016, from http://worlddatabaseofhappiness.eur.nl/hap_quer/introtext_measures5.pdf.

Veenhoven, R. (2016a). *World database of happiness*. Erasmus University Rotterdam, the Netherlands. Retrieved February 25, 2016, from http://worlddatabaseofhappiness.eur.nl.

Veenhoven, R. (2016b). *Measures of happiness, world database of happiness*. Erasmus University Rotterdam, The Netherlands. Retrieved February 25, 2016, from http://worlddatabaseofhappiness.eur.nl/hap_quer/hqi_fp.htm.

Ventegodt, S. (1995). *Quality of life in Denmark. Results from a population survey*. Copenhagen, Denmark: Forskningcentrets Forlag.

Watson, D., Clark, L. A., & Tellegen, A. (1988). Development and validation of brief measures of positive and negative affect: The PANAS scales. *Journal of Personality and Social Psychology, 54*(6), 1063–1070.

Weijters, B., Cabooter, E., & Schillewaert, N. (2010). The effect of rating scale format on response styles: The number of response categories and response category labels. *International Journal of Research in Marketing, 27*(3), 236–247.

Weng, L. J. (2004). Impact of the number of response categories and anchor labels on coefficient alpha and test-retest reliability. *Educational and Psychological Measurement, 64*(6), 956–972.

Wessman, A. E., & Ricks, D. F. (1966). *Mood and personality*. Oxford, England: Holt, Rinehart, & Winston.

White, A. (2007). A global projection of subjective well-being: A challenge to positive psychology? *Psychtalk, 56*, 17–20.

Winkelmann, L., & Winkelmann, R. (1998). Why are the unemployed so unhappy? *Evidence from panel data. Economica, 65*(257), 1–15.

Wright, T. A., & Cropanzano, R. (2004). The role of psychological well-being in job performance: A fresh look at an age-old quest. *Organizational Dynamics, 33*(4), 338–351.

Wright, T. A., & Staw, B. M. (1999). Affect and favorable work outcomes: Two longitudinal tests of the happy—Productive worker thesis. *Journal of Organizational Behavior, 20*, 1–23.

WVS Association (World Values Survey Association). (2016). *World values survey* (website). Abgerufen unter: http://www.worldvaluessurvey.org. zuletzt abgerufen am June 10, 2015.

Kai Ludwigs is a studied Psychologist, studied Economist and Founder and Director of the Happiness Research Organisation. In his studies, he researches how constructs like happiness, well-being and quality of life can be measured more accurately using modern technologies. He is an international expert in the topics of well-being, positive psychology, time use and happiness. He is a Board member of the International Society for Quality of Life Studies (ISQOLS) and the International Association for Time Use Research (IATUR).

Lena Henning is a psychologist focusing on measurements for happiness, subjective well-being and quality of life. During her time at the Happiness Research Organisation she worked on well-being assessment systems for cities, corporates and individuals.

Lidia Arends is professor of Methodology and Statistics at the Department of Psychology, Education, and Child Studies (DPECS), Erasmus University Rotterdam, The Netherlands. She also works as a biostatistician at the Department of Biostatistics, Erasmus MC, Rotterdam, the Netherlands. Her research focuses mainly on the statistical aspects and applications of (multi-variate) meta-analysis in social sciences as well as in medical science. Her work is highly cited, especially the "Tutorial on advanced statistical methods for meta-analysis" written together with Van Houwelingen and Stijnen in 2002 is used/cited more than 700 times (Web of Science).

Chapter 2
An Indigenous Perspective on Quality of Life

Pat Lauderdale

> *There is a big difference between living well and those who believe that living well is to live better than someone else. This latter view reflects a competition instead of respect and equality. Yet, 'living well' is the exercise of rights, respect, equality, and means a life for everyone.*
>
> —Blanca Chancoso

Abstract The substantive reliance on the interrelatedness of nature is one of the most interesting features of indigenous peoples. Current requests for global diversity and higher forms of the quality of life are indeed limited when they are built within the constraints of modern nation-states, which often views diversity as deviance if it does not conform to modern norms and definitions. Traditional indigenous knowledge has the potential for long-lasting approaches to current environment problems and provide us with ideas on how to improve our questions and, therefore, improve our potential for more equitable, less oppressive structures from which to approach the numerous problems. Indigenous Peoples with traditional perspectives and actions can provide us with significant paths to diversity throughout our planet, similar to the so-called ecological system. Internal colonialism and generations of domination create deep complications; therefore, the roles and actions of traditional peoples are central to our future and the generations to come. We can learn that the point is not to simply focus, for example, upon human rights and an anthropocentric sense of keeping things natural or simply being against pollution, but more upon the respect for and learning from nature by traditional indigenous peoples.

This chapter is an extension of the continual research on indigenous law-ways with Barbara Grey Kanatiiosh who helped initiate the ideas, and a revision of "Indigenous Peoples in the Face of Globalization." I would like to thank Karen Cook and the Institute for Research in the Social Sciences at Stanford University, and the School of Social Transformation at ASU and Elsie Moore for supporting this work. I also thank Ron Anderson who provided thoughtful comments on earlier drafts that were very helpful.

P. Lauderdale (✉)
Wilson Hall, 271, Tempe, AZ 85287-4902, USA
e-mail: pat.lauderdale@asu.edu

© Springer Nature Switzerland AG 2019

Y. Kee et al. (eds.), *Perspectives on Community Well-Being*, Community Quality-of-Life and Well-Being, https://doi.org/10.1007/978-3-030-15115-7_2

Keywords Indigenous people · Indigenous knowledge · Quality of life · Globalization

2.1 Prologue

Wolves are crucial for maintaining a healthy ecosystem—a fact that was conveniently forgotten when they were exterminated from almost all the continental United States by ranchers, farmers, trappers and hunters. Meanwhile, the populations of other animals exploded. The entire ecosystem of the American wilderness was changed by rapidly expanding populations of large ungulates.

After decades of political wrangling with those who traditionally persecuted wolves, conservation biologists and activists who supported restoration of wolves finally prevailed: the grey wolf, Canis lupus, was finally reintroduced several areas in the northern Rocky Mountains of the United States. One of those release areas was Yellowstone National Park. Subadult wolves from several packs in Alberta's Mackenzie Valley were captured using tranquilizer darts and released in Yellowstone in January 1995 and again in January 1996.

After an absence of nearly 70 years, the beneficial influences of the reintroduced wolves almost immediately became apparent and continue to be seen to this day. Since they are apex predators that primarily hunt ailing and aging ungulates—particularly wapiti, Cervus canadensis, whose populations had exploded in Yellowstone—wolves halted these herbivores' population expansions whilst improving their overall health (These animals are more commonly known as "elk" —note that the narrator in the accompanying video erroneously refers to these animals as "deer", implying that they are European red deer, Cervus elaphus, which they most certainly are not).

The presence of wolves even substantially changed ungulate behaviors. For example, the wapiti stopped munching their way through the valleys and gorges where wolves could easily ambush them. Thus, native flora was able to re-establish and re-grow, thereby increasing biodiversity by providing food and shelter to a growing variety of plants and animals.

But remarkably, the presence of wolves also changed the rivers. After reintroduction, it was noticed that riverbank erosion decreased so the rivers meandered less, the channels deepened and small pools formed. Why? The recovering vegetation stabilized the riverbanks, which in turn altered the geography of the park itself.

Basically, humans conducted a huge real-life experiment by removing—and then eventually reintroducing—an apex predator from a large tract of land. Initially, the ecological changes wrought by the lack of wolves were subtle so they were not generally noticed. But the results of this real-life reintroduction experiment unambiguously indicate that wolves are an integral part of the ecosystem; they certainly are essential to restoring and maintaining the natural ecology of the entire Yellowstone region.

This phenomenon is known amongst ecologists as a "trophic cascade". In this scenario, a top-down cascade was observed when the top predator, the wolf, was exterminated from most of its natural range. Removing the top predator triggered a

wide range of effects that cascaded down through the entire web of life. Although only a total of 41 wolves were reintroduced and their total population remains small, they act as ecosystem engineers by creating niches that other animal and plant species can inhabit (GrrlScientist Maniraptora, 2014).

A common ground for traditional indigenous peoples stems from their respect for all life forms rather than the modern separation of humans from the environment. From a traditional indigenous perspective, we cannot take a walk in nature because we are part of nature. Nature is not something separate from us. Esteva suggests that among traditional indigenous peoples, everyday life is more about learning than receiving an education and focuses more upon healing rather than dominating the environment or body. From a traditional perspective, no one can learn for you or heal you. Taking charge of learning instead of being educated, or of healing rather than being cured, reflects the continuous exercise of dignity and autonomy that characterizes most traditional indigenous peoples.

In contrast, most contemporary individuals have been taught that the environment is external to them, and that the human (animal) has the right to control the environment solely for its ends. This anthropocentric perspective attempts to control and dominate nature, that is, people and all forms of environment (Nader, 2002). Despite the recent discovery that the Greeks were concerned about environmental damage a few thousand years ago, their varied response to protecting it remains vague. Recent social control, for example, in the form of new laws and related social regulations that intend to protect the environment are usually shortsighted and fragmented, and often focus upon modern notions of developing the environment. Most ostensible developers attempt to control and dominate nature and then define this process as progress. Rather than learning the diverse lessons of nature via traditional indigenous peoples, the modern linear, univariate global development plan attempts to control and dominate nature, including rainforests, food sources, animals/humans or natural technologies (Lauderdale & Gray Kanatiiosh, 2007; Phillips & Wharton, 2015).

2.2 Globalization and the Quality of Life

Globalization is a series of economic, cultural and political changes typically viewed as increasing interdependence, integration and interaction between people and organizations throughout the world (Cruit & Lauderdale, 2016). The current dominant view of the process claims that it is a change that brings an increased standard of living and prosperity to poor countries and further wealth to rich ones. A critical perspective suggests that globalization is primarily another form of corporate imperialism that violates the rights of poor or marginalized peoples, and often perpetuates the long history of plundering and profiteering. This view focuses upon forced cultural assimilation, the export of artificial demands both material and symbolic, and the destruction or inhibition of local and global democracy along with the erosion of community, ecology and cultures.

Indigenous peoples have been resisting the negative phases of globalization for centuries in the western hemisphere, and for millennia in Africa and Eurasia. (Fenelon and Hall, 2005). Globalization is a process that is deeply connected to the first invention of states, at least, over 5000 years ago (Oliverio & Lauderdale, 2015). Fenelon and Hall emphasize that although social movements and protests based on indigenous perspectives concerning the negative aspects of globalization have changed over time, typically they are not interested in reforming the world system. They are more interested in autonomy and collective-determination, or what is termed self-determination in modern times. And, traditional indigenous forms of law or law-ways are central to autonomy and collective-determination (Pommersheim, 1995).

A central reason that law in modern societies is fundamentally different than the law of many traditional indigenous peoples is because the jurisprudence created by the modern nation-state assumes that law and nature should be separated. In contrast, a common feature of indigenous cultures based on traditional perspectives, however, is that law and nature are bound together. In indigenous cultures, for example, what is now termed law is not considered to be contained within the realm of nation-state structures, autonomous from other social relationships, interpreted only by legal specialists whose primary function is punishment as a means of state control and political legitimacy.

Indigenous forms of law are relatively direct and accessible to indigenous peoples since they are based on concrete notions of the individual and collective good rather than modern abstractions imposed by the nation-state as the ideal to which people must conform (or be punished) in order to have stability, security and individual material goods. For most traditional indigenous peoples, law is accessible to everyone since the oral tradition allows it to be carried around as part of them rather than confined to legal institutions (Lauderdale, 1997). Oral traditions in indigenous life stimulate, develop, protect and deliver knowledge in a systemic manner and jurisprudence based on oral traditions has continued to preserve much of the diversity and respect for nature. In his work with North American indigenous peoples, Vine Deloria suggests that within the traditions, beliefs, and customs of the peoples are the guidelines for preserving life and the future of all nature. Peoples are instructed to learn from nature rather than try to control and "develop" it for various ends (Deloria, 1992). Many indigenous groups in the Americas were initially viewed as "nations" by European "immigrants," and accorded varying degrees of autonomy and rights. As the Eurocentric ideas came to dominate, there were repeated efforts to transform indigenous nationhood into a minority status (Hall & Fenelon, 2005). Colonialism also sought to transform indigenous law-ways claiming they were too simplistic and should be based on Eurocentric versions of reason.

Colonization throughout the world was reflected in the creation of simplistic images of indigenous people as either primitive or dangerous. Those labels denied the complexity associated with diverse indigenous cultures. And, modern claims of progress and civilization as part of the domination of nature is conjecture, as is the imposition of backward and primitive to nature. In this context, the term primitive is a result of different types of ethnocentrism derived from narrow enlightenment philosophies and the concept of nature becomes a conundrum—nature has never been backward.

Most dominant philosophical traditions, however, continue to emphasize "the state of nature" as separate from humans in order to dominate nature. And the issue of human nature often turns into questions about race or utopian naturalism. Pseudospeciation, a human and modern invention that leads people to define their own species as another in order to extinguish life for narrow political and economic purposes, is not a lesson taken from nature. In contrast, from an indigenous perspective, Deloria (1992) notes that "if all things are related the unity of creation demands that each life form contribute its intended contribution. Any violation of another entity's right to existence in and of itself is a violation of the nature of creation and a degradation of religious reality itself" (299). The care for and examination of nature provides the lessons that can demonstrate the relevance and importance of diversity. A deep understanding of diversity contains ideas and methods of practicing responsibility and ensuring the existence of future generations.

Traditional indigenous knowledge of diversity is useful in adapting to change (Lyons, 1992). The saying that the only thing that is constant is change can be deeply understood from such a perspective. Traditional indigenous peoples know intimately that their histories were filled with adaptations and changes even long before colonization, and that evolution is not necessarily a positive word. Onomatopoeic research may provide insights into learning specific lessons from nature. Concerns about autonomy and collective-determination are deeply embedded in most indigenous oral history. And, a common issue is the collective responsibility for the nation and its resources, along with the concept of stewardship, as opposed to ownership (Fenelon & Hall, 2005; Hall & Fenelon, 2005).

Indigenous knowledge, which emerges from a symbiotic relationship between nature and underlying transformations, can continue to help us learn more about restoration. This restoration includes all living things. An examination of many indigenous societies shows us that struggles to achieve equality before efficiency is crucial and egalitarian policy solutions are essential Connerley and Wu (2015). Despite numerous attempts of holocaust proportion to destroy indigenous peoples, some of them and important parts of their traditional knowledge have persisted (Rodriguez & Lauderdale, 2014). Cultural values and social organization based on learning the lessons of nature are central to this persistence. Moreover, issues concerning the relatively small size of most indigenous nations and their homogeneity are important considerations, yet, despite comparable size and homogeneity of numerous modern subcultures or similar groups, they typically do not possess the social organization or cultural values of the indigenous peoples who lived symbiotically with nature. Most scientists remain perplexed, for example, by the fact that they have not uncovered or discovered any jails or prisons in most indigenous places (Lauderdale, 1997; Oliverio and Lauderdale, 2005). Different indigenous peoples living in quite diverse cultures and speaking many different languages did not find such a lesson from learning about the complexities of nature.

One important issue about the quality of life concerns the kinship structure of many indigenous cultures. Ideas emerging from this structure are not used as a simple social technique or as a punitive moral standard for a nation. The ideas include a respect for diversity rather than only tolerance, and a critical examination of fundamental concepts such as individual responsibility, group rights, time, and nature. In contrast, the concepts of well-being and quality of life in current research often are constructed variously because of the use of not only different values and different research instruments but also reflecting differing standpoints, differing purposes, and differing theoretical views and ontological presuppositions (Fayers & Machin, 2016).

There are thousands of indigenous nations living within the less than 200 nation-states in the modern world. Hall and Fenelon (2005) note the error in claiming that indigenous peoples have been ignored because they are numerically small and because they are disappearing, and though that hegemonic facade has been made for several hundred years, the numbers of indigenous peoples are actually growing. Indigenous people comprise from five to six percent of the world's population. Hall and Fenelon (2005) also point out that this number is approximately the equivalent of the United States or Europe, yet their influence and impact on global processes extend well beyond their numbers. Part of the reason is because indigenous peoples are beset with problems that many people take for granted, including free expression of language and religion, the right to live within self-determined cultures and traditions, and basic sustenance such as clean water, air, and land. Increasingly, indigenous nations throughout the world are courted by developers who want to ostensibly modernize them by establishing economic incentives via waste disposal companies, mining corporations, energy producers and other development schemes that have proven in the past to be polluting and often deadly to the environment. Non-indigenous communities often reject similar proposals to develop since they do not want to pollute their own backyards.

The thrust of neoliberalism and most development is economic reductionism, which seeks to place the economic market as first and foremost as it reduces local citizen power (Hanson, 2002). Hanson notes the historically imposed vulnerabilities that colonialism has placed upon indigenous peoples and explains how housing forms of garbage, including nuclear waste, on indigenous lands is similar to the methods factories use in poor countries when those companies attempt to avoid environmental, labor and related regulations. Moreover, he points out that for developers and most business people, time is money, however, for indigenous peoples' time may be more important for consensus. Consensus often is more important that material gains. Hanson also notes that traditional Dakotas' remark that everything comes from the earth and only recently was something invented by human animals that threaten everything that lives on this earth. Those indigenous peoples suggest that the nuclear threat was created by a society that claimed it was quite civilized and not primitive. For many indigenous peoples the current problem may be how to embrace the tar baby of new global capitalism as a means of economic self-determinations but not let that step become the thing itself, not let economic development become the predominant justification (Hanson, 2002).

Hanson also explicates that contemporary global warming is a human induced phenomenon, triggered by the burning of fossil fuels, which are products of millions of years of bio-diversity gathered in varied places in the earth. Fossil fuels are the concentrated carbon from plants and animals that lived over the hundreds of millions of years that life has been active. These fossils are burned for modern "wants" (not necessarily needs), including our sources of energy, transforming the liquid and solid carbon deep in the earth into air–born carbon and released into our atmosphere. Global warming is the end result of the use of those fossils over the last couple hundred years, particularly over the last half of the 20th century. Just as carbon is our largest single form of garbage, the most prodigious form of garbage in modern times, our atmosphere is our largest single garbage dump.

In general, people have much less access to the means of production, and dependency on scarce and underpaid work increases. Destruction of the welfare state also erodes the tradition whereby people could rely on the community to provide for them in times of crisis. During the early stages of privatization, services and products appeared to be less expensive; however, increasingly the terms of exchange shift, and most people have to rely on private services that are often much worse in quality, are typically less reliable, and are now more expensive than public services, despite corporate claims to the contrary.

The recent reinvention of the "colonization of the world" is informed by the "long sixteenth century," when the conquest of the Americas, their exploitation and colonial transformation led to the rise and so-called "development" of Europe. Cultural, traditional and ecological considerations are being abandoned to the method of plundering for profit (see Mann 2005). From an indigenous perspective, the abstract wealth created for accumulation is the destruction of nature as concrete wealth. When such concrete wealth is spent, abstract wealth disappears as well. Abstract wealth is not real wealth, which will become obvious. The result appears to be a conundrum of wealth, primarily existing virtually or on accounts, leaving a "monoculture" controlled by a few executives of multinational corporations. Diversity will be suffocated further or destroyed, with millions of people on the edge of survival. The neoliberal stranglehold also is creating a crisis of spirit that accompanies the material crisis. The annihilation of matter through its transformation into some type of commodity becomes more evident throughout the world.

2.3 Collective Rights Versus Human Rights

Evidence from traditional indigenous peoples suggest that acceptance of human rights and global diversity is indeed limited when it is built within the constraints of current law and narrow meanings of diversity, which often view development as deviance if it does not conform to modern ideas and definitions via neoliberalism. Neoliberalism is examined as extending far beyond the West, as a major force in the world system, which contains an ongoing, extensive, relatively complex social division of labor with an integrated set of production processes that are intimately related to the resources and lives of indigenous peoples throughout the world.

The spread of neoliberalism is deep and wide, and its scope runs far beyond the image of the West (Lauderdale & Natividad, 2010). And, examples from Dubai or Beijing are only the tip of the proverbial iceberg, or in this case the more obvious cutting-edge of the thrust. While the world press recently has spread the word of the trials and tribulations of the Tibetan people, most of the rest of the indigenous issues and peoples of the world are ignored, for example, those who continue to try to survive in Pakistan and Afghanistan. Peoples who typically are considered as indigenous such as the Sindhis and the Baluchi who reside or resided in Pakistan, Afghanistan and Iran are having their centuries old cultures eroded or destroyed by forces that are attached to the neoliberal movement. People who live along the Khyber Pass, the Phanthans (also called Pushtuns) who fought against the domination by the Chechens and Arabs continue resisting deadly intrusions from Pakistani and Afghan border troops. Ironically, the Kurram Agency of tribal areas of Pakistan usually is referred to as geography of tribal areas. Elders who have engaged for centuries in conflict negotiation such as the Jirga are increasingly redefined as old people who need to move along or aside.

Changes in the neoliberal thrust continue to be marginal. Global partnerships continue to be difficult to establish. Indigenous Peoples' representatives to the United Nations formally withdrew from the Working Group on Protected Areas of the Convention on Biological Diversity. They protested their exclusion from crucial meetings and wore symbolic gags and displayed protest signs. The Indigenous Women's Biodiversity Network warned that the exclusion of Indigenous Peoples not only endangers the democratic processes in the United Nations but also ignores that the General Assembly just approved the United Nations Declaration on the Rights of Indigenous Peoples. Human rights still maintain a focus on the Human animal rather than the diversity of our related living beings. And, the rarely mentioned role of covert international "security" agents who continue to portray themselves as working for human rights seriously erodes healthy relationships with traditional indigenous peoples.

Indigenous peoples throughout the world are experiencing the full presence of injustice in the form of duplicitous human rights agents, development schemes, poverty, landlessness, dispossession, political and religious oppression, and genocide. The indigenous peoples and their supporters resist the injustices, but resistance is only part of the struggle. People's Global Action (PGA), which is directly related to the Zapatista movement, calls for direct action and civil disobedience and the construction of local alternatives to the destruction of the environment and dominant economic relationships. The Zapatistas reflect a current manifestation of half a millennium of struggle with the Spanish, then the Mexican, and now global attempts to destroy indigenous peoples (Hall & Fenelon, 2005). The Zapatistas and the PGA reflect some of the diverse influences of their indigenous sources. Its website suggests that PGA is seen by some participants as an instrument for communication and coordination, not as an organization. It notes that it has no membership and no one can speak in its name. There is no leadership, although continental conveners can be periodically elected to organize conferences and maintain important communication tools. The diverse values and issues shared by the people in this movement emphasize their objections to rigid social hierarchies and the deadly results of such inflexibility.

Bruce Johansen (2003) has explicated cogently the terror indigenous peoples across the globe are facing in life-and-death struggles to maintain environments threatened by oil spills, explosions, toxic chemicals, global warming (potentially a real weapon of mass destruction), and other pollutants. Forms of resistance and ideas for social change can be found throughout the world. For example, the struggles against oil contamination by The Mapuche in Argentina; the plight of the indigenous peoples of Brazil concerning the problems of the rubber workers experienced by the followers of the late Chico Mendes; the fight against deforestation in the Congo Basin and Eritrea; the response to uranium poisoning in the Jharkand Belt in Bihar, India; and the responses to copper-mining spills experienced by the Marinduque Islanders in the Philippines. Social movements and organizations such as Cultural Survival, Greenpeace, Rainforest Action Network, and the World Wildlife Federation, engage in similar struggles against injustice and for nature. Of course, indigenous movements and environmental movements have crucial differences. The environmental movements increasing influenced by human rights concerns typically do not respond directly to indigenous issues and often promote the concept of the "empty" wilderness or nature park, that is, in contrast to movements that focus upon indigenous issues such as the Indigenous Environmental Network.

One of the most interesting features of indigenous peoples is their substantive reliance on the interrelatedness of nature. Today's call for, and acceptance of, global diversity and human rights is significantly limited when they are built within the constraints of modern nation-states, which often views diversity as deviance if it does not conform to modern norms and definitions. Traditional indigenous knowledge can't provide all the answers to current environment problems, however, it can provide us with ideas on how to improve our questions and, therefore, improve our potential to provide more equitable, less oppressive structures from which to approach the numerous problems.

When we couple political and economic conflicts with the intensifying conflict to control the Earth's dwindling natural resources, we make a general assessment that reflects a cloudy and troubled future. We appear to be living a schizophrenic existence; on one hand, we continue to make exciting discoveries that improve the general quality of life; on the other hand, we continue to live under conditions of immediate and mortal peril from our own lethal inventions and our voracious appetite to "consume." We have brought ourselves to a threshold of danger never before known in human history. Aside from the threat of weapons of mass destruction, our atmosphere is significantly polluted and falling apart, most of our forests are gone, most of our fresh water is poisoned, and with every passing day one or two species of animal or plant becomes extinct, with many more edging closer to doom. We need to stop what we're doing, take a deep breath and cast a critical eye on our most basic assumptions about all of existence on this Earth and our relationship to everything that lives here.

Peoples with traditional perspectives and actions provide us with the greatest diversity throughout our planet, similar to the so-called ecological system. They have the potential to give us the highest probability for future "foods" and symbiotic changes (cf. Phillips and Wharton, 2015). Internal colonialism and generations of domination create deep complications; therefore, the roles and actions of traditional peoples are central to our future and the generations to come. We can learn that the point is not to simply focus upon an anthropocentric sense of keeping things natural or simply being against pollution, but more upon the respect for and learning from nature by traditional indigenous peoples. The lesson from the wolves is just one example of learning the lessons of nature.

References

Connerley, M., & Wu, J. (2015). *Handbook on well-being of working women*. New York: Springer.

Cruit, M., & Lauderdale, P. (2016). *Globalogy and hegemony: A critical perspective* (2nd ed.). Phoenix, AZ: SRI Press.

Deloria, V., Jr. (1992). *God is red* (2nd ed.). Golden, CO: North American Press.

Fayers, P., & Machin, D. (2016). *Quality of life: The assessment, analysis and reporting of outcomes*. New York: Wiley-Blackwell.

Fenelon, J. V., & Hall, T. D. (2005). Indigenous struggles over autonomy, land and community: Anti-globalization and resistance in world systems analysis. In R. Grosfoguel, N. Maldonado-Torres, & J. David Saldivar (Eds.), *Latin@s in the world-system: Decolonization struggles in the 21st century U.S. Empire* (pp.107–122). Boulder: Paradigm Press.

GrrlScientist, Maniraptora. (2014, March 3). How wolves change rivers. *The Guardian*.

Hall, T., & Fenelon, J. (2005). Indigenous peoples and hegemonic change: Threats to sovereignty or opportunities for resistance? In J. Friedman & C. Chase-Dunn (Eds.), *Hegemonic decline: Present and past* (pp. 205–225). Boulder: Paradigm Press.

Hanson, R. D. (2002). Half lives of Reagan's Indian policy: Marketing nuclear waste to American Indians. *American Indian Culture and Research Journal, 25*(1), 21–44.

Johansen, B. (2003). *Indigenous peoples and environmental issues*. Westport, CT: Greenwood Press.

Lauderdale, P. (1997). Indigenous North American jurisprudence. *International Journal of Comparative Sociology, 38,* 131–148.

Lauderdale, P., & Gray Kanatiiosh, B. (2007). The great circle of justice: North American indigenous justice and contemporary restoration programs. *Contemporary Justice Review, 10*(2): 215–225.

Lauderdale, P., & Natividad, N. (2010). Global indigenous rights and responses. In R. Denemark (Ed.), *The international studies compendium* (pp. 3036–3056). Oxford: Wiley-Blackwell.

Lyons, O. (1992). The American Indian in the past. In O. Lyons, J. Mohawk, V. Deloria, Jr., L. Hauptman, D. Grinde, Jr., H. Berman, C. Berkey, & R. Venables, foreword by Peter Matthiessen, preface by Daniel K. Imouye, *Exiled in the land of the free: Democracy, Indian nations, and the U.S. Constitution* (pp. 13–42). Santa Fe, NM: Clear Light Publications.

Mann, C. C. (2005). *1491: New revelations of the Americas before columbus*. New York: Knopf.

Nader, L. (2002). *The life of the law*. Berkeley, CA: University of California Press.

Oliverio, A., & Lauderdale, P. (2005). *Terrorism: A new testament*. ON, Canada: de Sitter Publications.

Oliverio, A., & Lauderdale, P. (2015). The world system according to Andre Gunder Frank: Hegemony and domination (Andre Gunder Frank's *Reorienting the 19th century*). *Journal of World-Systems Research, 21*(1).

Phillips, R., & Wharton, C. (2015). *Growing livelihoods: Local food systems and development*. New York: Routledge.

Pommersheim, F. (1995). *Braid of feathers: American Indian law and contemporary tribal life*. Berkeley, CA: University of California Press.

Rodriguez, P., & Lauderdale, P. (2014). Hegemony and collective memories: Japanese American relocation and imprisonment on American Indian "Land." In S. Bowman (Ed.), *Color behind bars: Racism in the U.S.* (pp. 119–133). Santa Barbara, CA: ABC-CLIO, Greenwood Press.

Pat Lauderdale holds a Ph.D. from Stanford University, and is Professor of Justice and former Director of the University-wide Ph.D./J.D. program in Justice Studies, Law, and the Social Sciences at ASU. His teaching and research interests include comparative law, indigenous jurisprudence, racialization, diversity, global indigenous struggles, and international terrorism. He is author or coauthor of numerous books, including *Lives in the Balance, Terrorism: A New Testament, Theory and Methodology of World Development, The Struggle for Control: A Study of Law, Disputes and Deviance,* and *Law and Society*, Japanese translated version (Miyazawa), *Invitation to Globalogy*, and *A Political Analysis of Deviance, third edition.*

Chapter 3
A Participatory Process: Creating Child Friendly Environments

E. Ümran Topcu and Sebnem Cana Kacar

Abstract Cities compose of heterogeneous populations with different needs. Needs of the "children" portion of urban populations has not been examined enough, according to study at hand, in Turkey. Popularity of the cities seems to be increasing and people tend to move to urban areas rather than suburban. The case happens to be the same in Turkey, like elsewhere in the world. Especially in İstanbul Turkey, after 1950s there happened a rapid migration ending in rapid urbanization. İstanbul got the biggest piece out of internal migration combining into factors that end in an environment not friendly for children. Over the last 10 years or so, interest in the child friendly cities has increased in Turkey along with the rest of the developed world for two main reasons: (1) 2008 was the first time more people started to live in urban areas; and (2) there is a worldwide trend towards government decentralization. However, local authorities were not prepared to respond due to limited resources. This chapter explores children's existing environment in a specific locale in İstanbul, in order to transform it into a child friendly one. There are some aspects that are elaborated such as; mobility of children in city centers, everyday life of children, children's involvement in planning decisions. In the guideline of these issues, a design proposal is introduced in the end, which was discussed with the residents of Akkirman Street in the Şişli district of İstanbul. The experiences and desires of children do have much to offer in planning practice and in turn it has much to teach children about citizenship, responsibility and participation.

Keywords Children · City · Participatory planning · Child friendly design

---

E. Ü. Topcu (✉) · S. C. Kacar
Bahçeşehir Üniversitesi, Kuzey Kampüsü, Mimarlık ve Tasarım Fakültesi, Abbasağa Mahallesi, Ihlamur Yıldız Caddesi No. 8, 34353 Beşiktaş, İstanbul, Turkey
e-mail: umran.topcu@arc.bau.edu.tr

S. C. Kacar
e-mail: sebnem.kacar@gmail.com

© Springer Nature Switzerland AG 2019

Y. Kee et al. (eds.), *Perspectives on Community Well-Being*, Community Quality-of-Life and Well-Being, https://doi.org/10.1007/978-3-030-15115-7_3

3.1 Introduction

> Cities have the capability of providing something for everybody, only because and only when they are created by everybody.

This famous quote by Jane Jacobs (1961), leads everyone to take part in the design process of the city they are part of. Actually, most planning practices exclude children even though there is growing body of research that shows how and why they could and should participate (Checkoway, 1998; Ginwright & James, 2002; O'Donoghue, Kirshner, & McLaughlin, 2002). In some few cases where children are included in the planning practice, it is often only intertwined with considerations of all residents, with no special consideration of the needs and voices of children (Knowles-Yanez, 2005). Is it because childhood is considered as a temporary stage of life? Childhood is a very special and fragile stage of life according to the specialists. Introducing children to decision making helps educating them early on responsibilities and enhancing their capacity of being responsible citizens. As it stands in most parts of the world, they are invisible in decision making or planning processes. Besides historical conceptualizations of childhood, reasons are likely:

- Assumptions of parties who have interest in planning
- Laws and regulations about the use of urban space being seen as adult's topics

Although children represent a large group in city population they are still considered as not important assets in urban design process. A child-friendly city points out that the city is a platform to lead children to be important in supporting the physical and social development of their city. Having a relationship, self-expression and socializing are primary needs of any individual since early childhood. These are not important only for building a healthy mental and social future for children, but also considered as equally important for a progressive urban space. The existence of a friendly urban space depends on the degree of people's comfort, mobility, freedom and motivation in that city.

The city is a social product, so it is crucial to address a problem of creating any designed environment by means of a thorough understanding of life that takes place in it. The city with all its locales should be a place to make children feel safe and comfortable in the physical sense and the symbolic sense. Well-designed urban areas should transmit equal messages both to children and the adults as equal members of the community.

3.2 Aim and Scope

In this study, questions like "What do the children need in their everyday life and cannot have?" and "Can an immediate environment be changed according to children's and parents' needs and wants?" are taken as primary concerns and according to the opinion survey done in the Şişli district of İstanbul.

How and what does it mean to involve children in planning research and practice? In a qualitative review of most international research and publication that are indicative of planning activities that involve children, four approaches are identified: scholarly, practice, educational and right-based approaches. Although borders between these approaches are porous, scholarly and educational approaches seems like they overlap. The practice approach has broad applications (Knowles-Yanez, 2005). Review of these approaches suggests future directions for children's participation in planning processes. Checkoway, Pothukuchi, and Finn (1995) propose scholarly and practice approaches, including accepting the involvement of children, as the correct and recommended action.

Both scholarly and educational approaches are not involved in this research. However, both of the approaches are setting children's mind free and creating a platform for brain storming. A strong supporter of scholarly approach is Moore (1990) saying that the importance of play in the natural physical environment develops a sense of environmental competence in children. There are other researchers who suggest different media in surveying the opinions of children, such as photography, dramatic improvisations, youth conferences and design workshops. These are seen as ways of involving children in remaking their local environments (Corbishley, 1995; Dierkx, 2003; Pancer, Rose-Krasnor, & Loiselle, 2002; Plester, Richards, Blades, & Spencer, 2002).

The right-based approach lets children to know about land-use planning and how their participation in decisions will affect their lives. The emphasis is on the roles of the children's voices in shaping their living environments (Bartlett, 2005; Chawla, 2002). The 1989 United Nations General Assembly Convention on the Rights of Children (RCR) is the most significant legal indication of this view. The CRC is central to many of the rights-based approaches to involving children in land use planning because it provides a framework by which to consider the rights of children. The document had a great impact on governmental level in every country in the world, except for Sudan.

Obviously, rights based approach in planning brought about the possibility of learning from children how they evaluate the places where they live and how they would like to live and then use this dialogue to bring children and adults together in participatory programs to improve the urban environments.

The idea behind participatory design is to systematically combine interdisciplinary theory and applications and involve the people in the planning and design phases of their surroundings. In addition to the benefits of people having the chance to actively take part instead of passively accept what is given, this process plays the important role of giving people that feeling of having been listened to. Thus, the planning activity itself becomes a learning process for both the designers and the inhabitants (Sanoff, 1990).

Roger Hart in his book *Children's Participation* (1997) has explained how people working with children might interpret the CRC by focusing on the authentic participation of children and action research with children. Most of his action research is executed outside the United States. He is in favor of the action research process in which children define the problem topic. He uses children as a mode of communication to publicize the problem issues and the children's authentic participation. According to the rights-based approach, children must be asked what suits them and adults should not assume they know what is best for children. Children are keen on the following conditions: convergence, entry for all to participate, social support, being seen as competent beings able to solve problems and producing results and reflection, negotiation, evaluation and understanding.

The theoretical base and the method for this study are founded on the specifications discussed previously of rights-based approach explained by Hart. As for the local factors prevailing in the chosen İstanbul locale, the below titles should be explained: mobility, psychological and social causes of restricted mobility and climate.

3.3 Mobility

Most of the parents residing in the Akkirman Street are part of the labor force and their working hours are between 8.00 am and 18.00 pm. If a child's bed time is 21.00 pm there will not be enough quality time for the whole family to enjoy together on the weekdays. Modern parents may also like to rest, dine or watch T.V instead of spending time with their children on the one hand, which might be considered normal after working at least 8 h a day, on the other hand (Figs. 3.1 and 3.2).

The general practice in Turkey is, children stay with the relatives (grandparents, aunts, sisters etc.) while the parents are at work. Being taken care of by grandparents means not having enough energy transfer between the two parties and to canalization of children's energy into creative activities. In other words, most children who live in urban areas are stuck at home. There is not always a playground in the immediate surroundings, nor there are any streets closed to traffic. Even if there were, it is still risky for children to play outside by themselves because of some outer reasons. Parents tend towards holding a particular view of their children. They are considered as vulnerable, extremely precious, fragile, disease prone through dirt, cold and easily susceptible to bad influences. These facts scare parents and they feel insecure when let their children play outside. This is a reason why children cannot move independently in their neighborhood. Their mobility is restricted.

3.4 Psychological and Sociological Causes of Restricted Mobility

Children of 21st century are not as physically active as the previous years. Developments in technology are very fast and within this context, access to technology is getting easier. Most children, even from middle and low-income households are playing PC and video games at home or in internet cafes. Virtual games have taken over real games played with peers in the real world. Most parents seem to accept this situation because of their limited time and energy. The virtual world has been attracting both boys and girls alike. In 1990s the case was not the same because the accessibility to technology was not that easy and PC games attracted boys more than girls. Playing outside, visiting peers and playing interactive games, belonging to the real world were still popular back then. Today the case is different, now it is more attractive for children to play with a tablet, even when they are together with their friends they prefer to look at a screen. It is obvious that children are getting lonelier and more introverted with the help of modern urban world. Their communication skills are not improving and the question is what is going to happen in a not too distant future?

It is very important to solve this problem and maybe the solution is teaching the children: being social is a need, and communication is one of the most important assets in life. Also, there are some other facts we do not know yet which are about health. We do know that standing still and malnutrition caused obesity, and scientific studies show that: being involved with electronic devices causes cancer, we have not seen the most serious effects of this yet, however this is a process and the usage of electronic devices increased in last 10 years. Unfortunately, the side effects will be observed in the future.

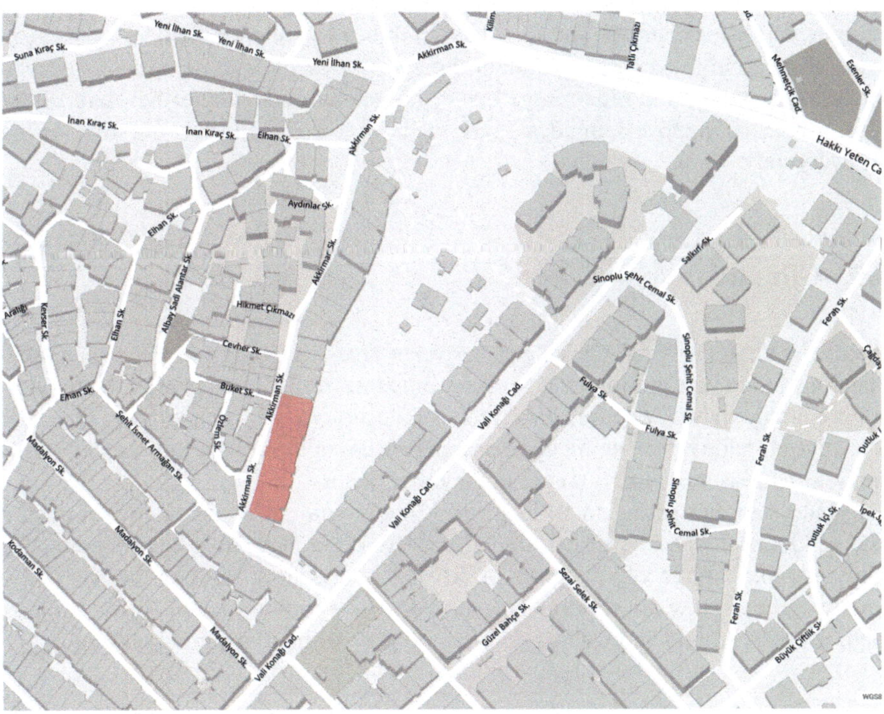

Fig. 3.1 The red area indicates the chosen buildings on Akkirman Street of Nişantaşı

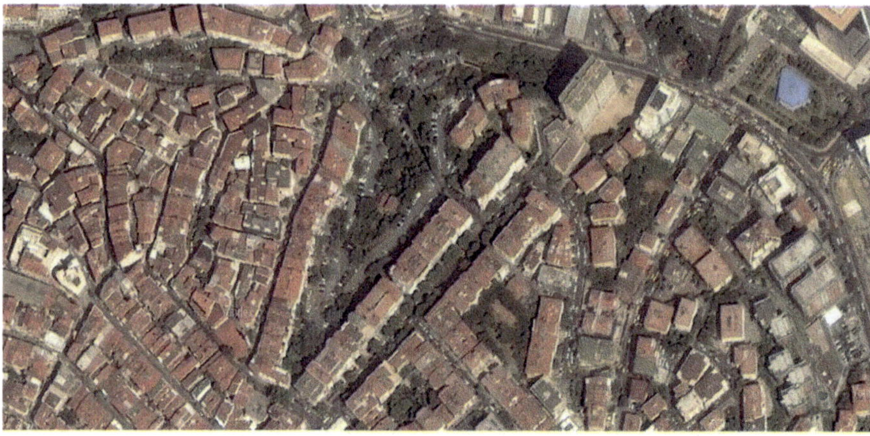

Fig. 3.2 Aerial view of Akkirman Street of Nişantaşı

Children need to be free and explore everything when they can. They need to interact with the nature, know about animals, street cats, dogs etc. and the best way to learn is by observing and interacting. Do the children of 21st century, who live in cities, have this chance? The restricted mobility of children is affecting them in many aspects. In this context, an environment as a base for these issues is needed for bringing youth and elders together in the same arena where they will all be comfortable and happy. Being designers, we have to create the best possible setting for everybody.

3.5 Climate

Claire Freeman (1995) suggests greener open areas in the city in her paper titled Planning and Play: Creating Greener Environments, for children to play freely without second thoughts. A consensus on this suggestion may be omnipresent but there is always climatic effect acting upon design process in the city. In the context of this study, climate is more important than the other factors.

Winter, fall and spring in İstanbul are usually cold and rainy. Children cannot play outdoors freely. There has to be alternative designs or other environments for everyone, like Jane Jacobs suggests. A city has to include something for everybody who lives there. How can children be happy when the parents look upset for bringing them to a playground and waiting for them to play while it is raining outside?

3.6 Design Proposal

The authors being familiar with the before mentioned locale (see Figs. 3.1 and 3.2) of Nişantaşı Akkirman Street knew about the problems that inhabitants of this street went through. So, they proceeded through observation and interrogation with the locals. Surveys and assessments were based on observations of the locale.

The design proposal was supposed to be in accordance with some important issues. First: it had to be in the close vicinity of the chosen neighborhood. Second: it had to be free from traffic. Third: it had to be an affordable and applicable design. Fourth and last but not least, it had to provide all the before mentioned aspects: a shelter, open space, attractions both for children and adults alike, safety and security, some elements of nature, utilities for resting and eating together.

As for an early architectural archetype, Le Corbusier's Unité d'Habitation in Marseille, France was a source of inspiration. Completed in 14 October 1952, the design was considered to be the first manifestation of a roof top environment suited to modern life. It was not only an apartment block accommodating housing, but including social facilities and also parking for cars and bicycles. The building stands on pillars so as to respect the streetscape and not block the circulation. Most of the social facilities were located on the rooftop. There is a playground, a nursery, a roof garden, a small swimming pool for children, a gymnasium, an open space for physical training, a 300 m sprinters' track and a solarium with a snack bar.

The idea of utilizing the rooftops was not new. New ways of conceptualizing the idea and putting into action was the objective of the authors. The roofs of seven apartment blocks on Akkirman Street/Nişantaşı/İstanbul/Turkey were chosen as a pilot study area. The reason to choose this place is, the buildings provide the necessary site for the design proposal. They are mostly attached buildings and this provided the chance to have this design on several buildings with similar number of levels, being seven or eight stories high (Fig. 3.3). Although the height parameter matched between the buildings, there were some illegal extensions in the form of terraces. One common advantageous feature to combine these buildings was that they all had flat roofs (see Figs. 3.4, 3.5 and 3.6).

The roof top design has five lanes. The outer lanes are the boundaries, which are planned as a jogging or walking areas (see Fig. 3.7). By setting this function on the outer lanes, a definite behavior setting was defined. Only the people who chose to walk in this area would use these lanes and children would not get closer to the outer railings. Railings exist between lanes because of the physical nature of the design, having alternative heights and waves. The inner lanes are designed to be circulation lanes. They direct the users to upper and lower levels of the design. Also, the main access points from the apartment blocks to the roof are from these lanes. The central lane is the widest lane. On this lane are the hobby gardens designed in the form of raised pots. The plants grown by the children will not be affected by weather conditions. There is also a cut-out part on this lane for children to have an exciting attraction point. The attraction comes in the form of a net which provides a safe surface for children to relax and play.

At the lower level there are closed areas, namely an eating and relaxing zone both for children and adults. There are two long tables for all parties to sit together as a community. The reason for not having several tables is for the creation of a social atmosphere by sitting together. Especially children will learn to communicate with their peers. It is also important for the parents to re-learn intergenerational communication, too. There is a white board or cinema screen (see Fig. 3.6) at one end and bean bags in front of them to create a cozier atmosphere. This zone can be used as a multipurpose area. Another zone is especially for children between 3 and 7 years of age. A playground is not designed on the roof top, due to the rule no. 1 of this design being for everybody, not only for children. Another concern was not to disturb the top floors dwellers with noise. This area is chosen for sand filling, both as insulation and a representation of nature. The children will have a chance to experience nature with a clean sandbox. As for the artistic activities, there is an empty white washed wall for children to design. Tables at proper height will let children to get involved in creative activities and everything that is not allowed at home (see Figs. 3.8 and 3.9). There are also softer seats in the form of bean bags for children to enjoy and relax. When they want to play a game with the group they can easily move the furniture by themselves and clear the area in order to prepare for games. The best part of this area is that adults and children can talk about old

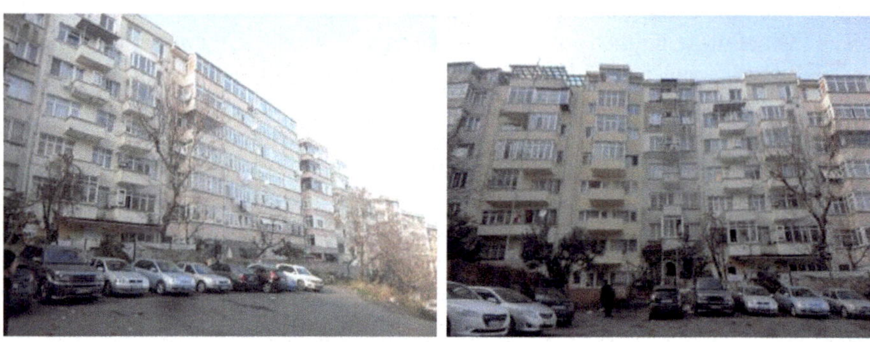

Fig. 3.3 Images showing the facades of the chosen apartment blocks

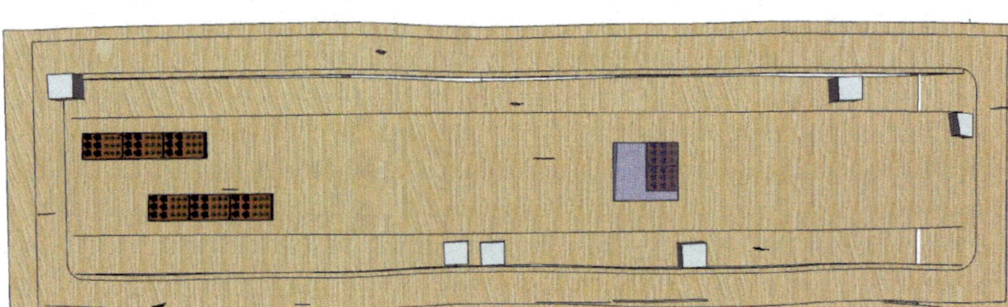

Fig. 3.4 Plan of the design proposal

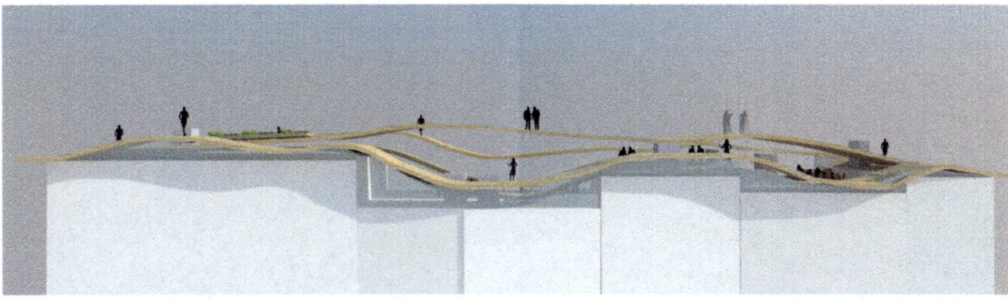

Fig. 3.5 Elevation of the design proposal

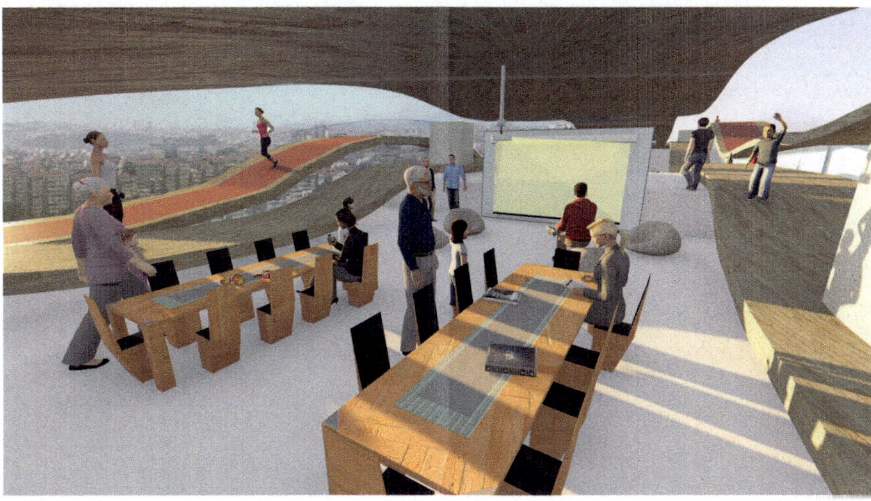

Fig. 3.6 Image showing an activity area

forgotten games that elders used to play on streets. This would be a nice platform for having stronger intergenerational relations. There is another hobby garden (see Fig. 3.10) under the central lane cut-out part. This garden is for the sensitive plants, which need to be kept from sunlight or cold.

3.7 Methodology

Participatory planning is an urban planning method that aims to engage and involve the community in the strategic and design process of a project. It is widely used in the design process of child friendly spaces, since it enhances the quality of the project by taking into consideration the insights of children, who will eventually be the users of the space. For the purpose of this study, a proposal started by talking to the local

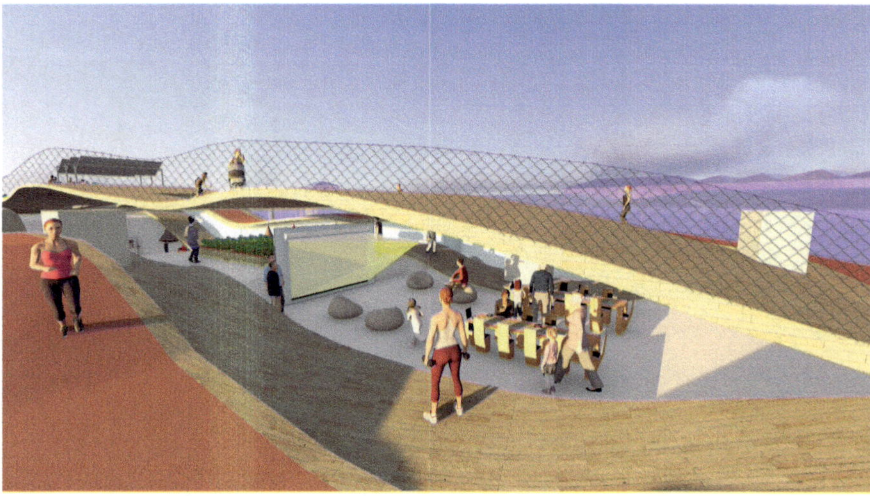

Fig. 3.7 Image showing the outer lanes

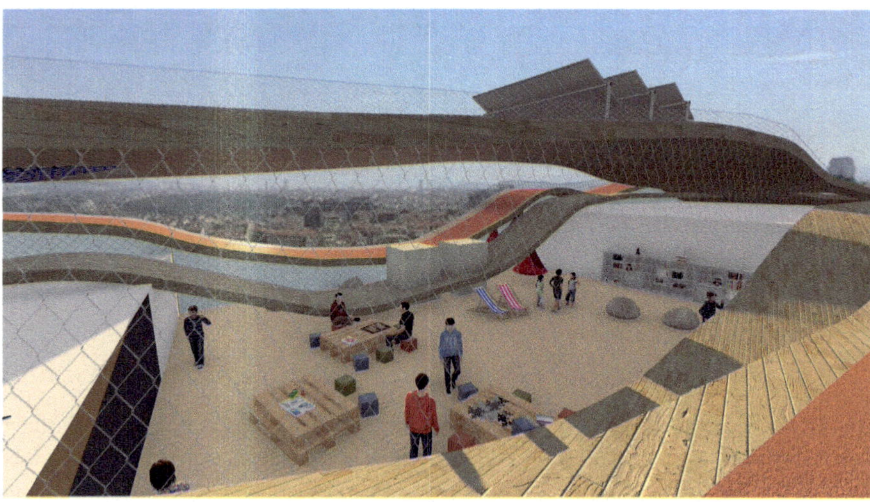

Fig. 3.8 Image showing the middle area

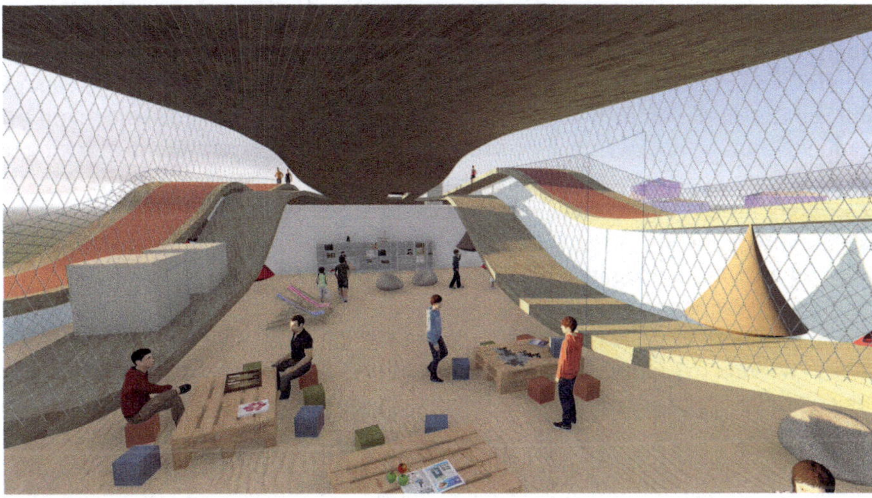

Fig. 3.9 Image showing an interaction area

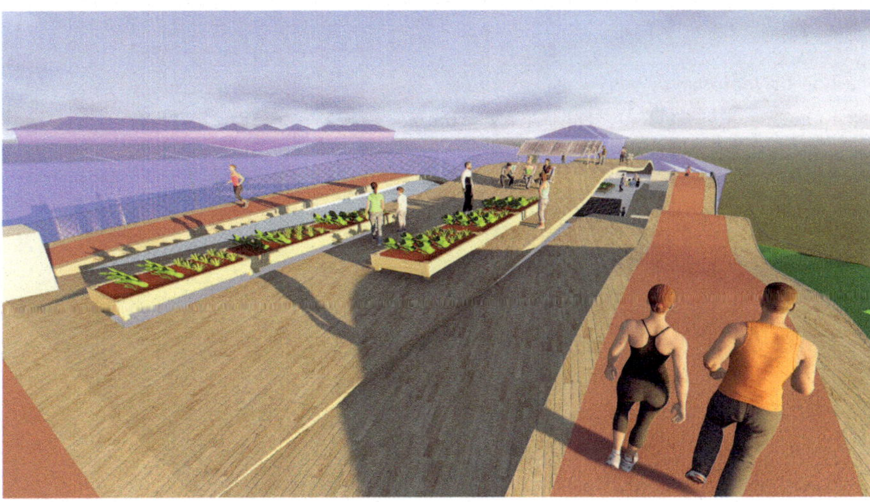

Fig. 3.10 Image showing the jogging lanes and the green area

people and especially asking children about their thoughts on the initiation of a child friendly immediate environment within their vicinity. A questionnaire composing of six questions were administered to the residents who lived in the chosen seven blocks of apartments. Due to time limitations it was not possible to use other techniques such as children's drawings, writings and behavior mapping, etc.

Interviews and meeting took place in the back yard. There happened to be only three non-residential units within the seven blocks, one of them being a dental clinic, and the other two offices of law firms. All the rest was residential; 75% of the parents were part of the labor force; and 80% of the residents were owners while only 20% were tenants. The participants' consensus was about not having enough public spaces in the immediate environment. Although they were satisfied with the location of their residence, several owners with children were considering moving to a gated community. They were not satisfied with security and social facilities. Mostly the working group complained about the lack of social facilities. Due to limited free time, they were not able to go somewhere for recreation. They all wished to have a facility of attraction in the immediate environment.

With few exceptions, children's thoughts were not different. The children between 7 and 12 years of age expressed their complaints of not being taken anywhere by their parents. Without exception, all were interested in outdoors. Most parents were over protective, they did not want to take them to the parks in central locales or woods because of the weather conditions. Even if they did, the time was limited and it could only happen only twice a month. Children between 3 and 6 years of age were not confident about their wishes, most probably due to lack of awareness. However, upon seeing the design proposal their mind set changed. The Questionnaire was organized around 6 questions and the following descriptive analysis ensued.

Question 1 (*How often do you take your children out?*)
31% of the parents took their children out ***few times a week***
29% of the parents took their children out ***everyday***
14% of the parents took their children out ***on alternate days***
5% of the parents took their children out ***few times a month***

Question 2 (*How satisfied are your children to participate activities out of the home?*)
38% of the children were ***satisfied***
32% of the children were ***very satisfied***
23% of the children were ***neither satisfied nor dissatisfied***
7% of the children were ***dissatisfied***

Question 3 (*Which is the most effective obstacle for you to go out for a different activity with children?*)
45% of the parents said there were ***no interesting activities in the immediate environment***
26% of the parents said they ***did not have enough time***
19% of the parents complained of ***lack of public transport***
10% of the parents complained of ***long distances***

Question 4 (*Where and for which purpose do you go out with your children most of the time?*)
42% to ***parks or playgrounds for recreation***
33% to ***malls for shopping***
21% to ***central areas for a difference***
2% to ***art galleries and museums for educational purposes***

Question 5 (*How effective would it be to have a social facility or green area in the immediate environment for you and your children?*)
48% said it would be ***effective***
24% said it would be ***very effective***
21% said it would be ***slightly effective***
7% said it would ***not be effective at all***

Question 6 (*What kind of qualities do you look for in a green area and/or social facility*)
29% look for ***open and semi open places***
26% look for ***secure places***
26% look for ***proximity***
19% look for ***variety of activities***

3.8 Conclusion

It was the opinion of the locals of Akkirman Street that they needed to improve their immediate environment for their children and themselves. The participatory planning process enabled the surfacing of residents both young and old, wishes and needs in a creative and participatory way.

In the beginning there was a rough idea and images about the design proposal, in the end of the meeting with locals, they were asked about their needs and wants, and the design proposal was designed according to that. The benefit of this study for the authors was, understanding the users as a designer. The meetings and interviews proved to be very promising, however other methods could have been used with children. Time limitation did not allow for more investigations, surveys or reaching more people. It would have been better to divide the users into age groups rather than talking to them all together. According to the observations, the actors were affected by each other's thoughts. Notably, children were impacted by their parents' ideas. A survey would have been a better technique for the adults and a meeting with children and asking them to draw pictures about their ideal environment would have been better methods. In general, workshops with children prove that they are skillful in expressing their feelings, wishes and criticisms by drawing, writing, making models or in other means if provided the opportunity.

One of the most crucial parts was the users' behaviors. They knew that they needed more common space, green area and social facilities, however they were not coming together for talking about this, even though the authors suggested for a meeting. It was very hard to bring all the users together and also the users were not enthusiastic to talk or even meet at the beginning. This was the hardest part of the study. In spite of the disadvantages and the imperfect methods, feedbacks were positive. In the end of this study it is understood that participatory planning is very hard without the willing actors. The actors are missing the most basic part of the process which is taking action.

Planning practice is charged with the task of helping people make decisions about how to use space. Those decisions usually contain complex indicators of interests from developers, citizens, and politicians. It is not an easy task to bring children's interests and rights forward into these processes. The experiences and wishes of children and adolescents have much to offer planning practice. At the same time, when they are involved they get the chance of learning about responsibility, citizenship, and participation.

References

Bartlett, S. (2005). Integrating children's rights into municipal action: A review of progress and lessons learned. *Children, Youth and Environments, 15*(2), 18–40.

Chawla, L. (2002). Insight, creativity and thoughts on the environment: Integrating children and youth into human settlement development. *Environment and Urbanization, 14*(2), 11–21.

Checkoway, B. (1998). Involving young people in neighborhood development. *Children and Youth Services Review, 20*(9/10), 765–795.

Checkoway, B., Pothukuchi, K., & Finn, J. (1995). Youth participation in community planning: what are the benefits? *Journal of Planning Education and Research, 14*(2), 134–139.

Corbishley, P. (1995). A parish listens to its children. *Children's Environments, 12*(4), 414–426.

Dierkx, R. (2003). Toward community-based architectural programming and development of inclusive learning environments in Nairobi's slums. *Children, Youth and Environments, 13*(1). http://colorado.edu/journals/cye.

Freeman, C. (1995). Planning and play: Creating greener environments. *Children's Environments, 12*(3), 381–388.

Ginwright, S., & James, T. (2002). From assets to agents of change: Social justice, organizing, and youth development. *New Directions in Youth Development, 96,* 26–27.

Hart, R. A. (1997). *Children's participation: The theory and practice of involving young citizens in community development and environmental care*. London: UNICEF.

Jacobs, J. (1961). *The death and life of American cities*. New York: Random House.

Knowles-Yanez, K. L. (2005). Children's participation in planning process. *Journal of Planning Literature, 20*(1).

Moore, R. C. (1990). *Childhood's domain: Play and place in child development*. Berkeley, CA: MIG Communications.

O'Donoghue, J. L., Kirshner, B., & McLaughlin, M. (2002). Introduction: Moving youth participation forward. *New Directions in Youth Development, 96,* 15–26.

Pancer, S. Mark, Rose-Krasnor, L., & Loiselle, L. D. (2002). Youth conferences as a context for engagement. *New Directions in Youth Development, 96,* 47–64.

Plester, B., Richards, J., Blades, M., & Spencer, C. (2002). Young children's ability to use aerial photographs as maps. *Journal of Environmental Psychology, 22*(1/2), 29–47.

Sanoff, H. (1990). *Participatory design*. Mansfield, OH: Bookmasters Inc.

E. Ümran Topcu is a Professor at Bahçeşehir University, Faculty of Architecture and Design, Istanbul, Turkey. She is a senior lecturer at the Faculty of Architecture and Design of Istanbul Bahcesehir University. Her Masters' degree is from the Istanbul State Academy of Fine Arts (1977) and her PhD from Istanbul Technical University, Department of Urban and Regional Planning (2004). She worked as a design architect at C.I.E Consulting Engineers in London (1982–1983), and in Riyadh as a lecturer and advisor for Al Nahda Philantrophic Society (1984–1995). She taught at Istanbul Beykent University, School of Architecture (1998–2003); since 2004, Topcu teaches Basic Design, Architectural Design Studies, People and Environment and Architectural Research Methodology at Istanbul Bahcesehir University Faculty of Architecture and Design. Topcu's areas of interest are architectural design, architectural education, people and environment, neighborhood and quality of life. She has contributed to the *Encyclopedia of Quality of Life and Well-Being* published by Springer and coordinated the International Summer and Winter Workshops between UPC ETSAB and BAU FA&D, held in Barcelona and Istanbul since 2012. She has a special interest in reading, writing, sketching and travelling.

Chapter 4
Community Well-Being and Migration Intention of Residents

YeonKyeong Lee and Seung Jong Lee

Abstract Korea is concerned with population declines, and the impact on overall well-being at the local level needs to be considered. This chapter provides a review of a study aimed at determining intention of residents to keep living within current communities by examining the influence of community characteristics on migration intention. This study tried to analyze the objective characteristics of the community through the distinction between urban and rural areas with different population sizes, structure, and economic characteristics. It was found that the objective characteristics of the community affected migration intentions.

Keywords Migration · Population decline · Community characteristics

4.1 Introduction

Today, South Korea (hereafter, Korea) is experiencing population problems. The population is decreasing due to low fertility and aging is rapidly progressing. Korea had a population of 25.01 million in 1960, 30 million in 1967, 40 million in 1983, and showed rapid population growth, reaching 50 million in 2012. However, this population growth is not expected to last long because the population will continue to decline after peaking in 2030 due to the unprecedented rapid decline in fertility rate (Ko & Huh, 2015).

In addition, Korea is experiencing the most rapid changes of structure of population due to low fertility and aging. As a result, in 2000, the proportion of the population over 65 years old exceeded 7% and has entered an aging society in earnest. As of 2018, the elderly population aged 65 or older reached 14.3%, becoming an aged society.

Y. Lee · S. J. Lee (✉)
Graduate School of Public Administration, Seoul National University, 1 Gwanak-ro, Gwanak-gu, Seoul 151-742, South Korea
e-mail: slee@snu.ac.kr

Y. Lee
e-mail: faloredo@hanmail.net

© Springer Nature Switzerland AG 2019
Y. Kee et al. (eds.), *Perspectives on Community Well-Being*, Community Quality-of-Life and Well-Being, https://doi.org/10.1007/978-3-030-15115-7_4

Above all, the pace of aging is so rapid that in 2050, the proportion of elderly people over 65 years old is expected to be the world's oldest, rising to 38.2% (Ko & Huh, 2015). Population decline and aging are worrying in that they can cause social and economic problems by lowering economic vitality and productivity, and raising welfare and social costs.

However, population decline and aging can have even more serious consequences at the local level. Local governments are suffering not only from declining natural populations, but also from declining social populations. The impact of population decline and aging can vary from region to region due to regional migration. The smaller the population and the more aged, the faster the population decline and aging. Therefore, it is difficult to achieve balanced regional development, and the regional decline and polarization can deepen.

Therefore, local governments need to cope with the problem of population decline and are interested in policy efforts to prevent the outflow of local residents. For this reason, "migration intention", which means "intention to continue to live in the current area of local residents", may be an important issue for local governments.

The purpose of this study is to investigate the factors influencing the migration intention of local residents and to examine the effects and implications of community well-being as a determinant of residents. Can Community well-being be a key alternative to local governments to maintain local populations and to improve the quality of life and happiness of local residents at a time of population decline? That is the main research question of this study.

4.2 Population Problems in Korea

Population is a very important indicator of a country. Proper population size and a virtuous circle of population structure (sex ratio and age) determine national development and sustainability. However, Korea is now suffering from population problems such as low fertility and aging. According to a report by Statistics Korea (National Statistical Office), "Future Population Estimate: 2015–2065" released in 2016, the total population will increase until 2031, and then decline thereafter approximately up to 43.2 million people by 2065. The population growth rate is also expected to turn negative in 2032 and to fall to −1.03% by 2065.

It is expected that not only the size of the population will decrease but also the structure of the population will change. The working age population (population aged 15–64) is expected to peak to 37.63 million in 2016 and to decrease by more than 300,000 per year from the 2020s. The youth population (population aged 0–14) is expected to decline from 7.03 million in 2015 to 4.13 million in 2065. In contrast, the elderly population (population aged 65 or older) is expected to increase from 6.54 million in 2015 to over 10 million in 2025 and to 18.27 million in 2065. This phenomenon, where working age population and the proportion of youth population is decreasing and the proportion of elderly population is increasing, is accompanied by changes in total support costs and aging index. According to the United Nations' population estimates, population decline is expected to occur in some Organization for Economic Co-operation and Development (OECD) countries between 2015 and 2065. However, the rate and magnitude of the change is expected to be large in Korea.

Thus, what are the impacts of population size and structural change? Many previous studies have analyzed the impact of changes in population size and structure on the economy and society. First, changes in population size and structure of population affect the labor force, unemployment, and employment, and these changes cause the population's change again (Je, 2018). Specifically, population decline and aging have been shown to decrease labor force, savings rate, and rate of economic growth, to slow down personal consumption and corporate investment, and to increase welfare costs such as medical care (Kim, 2016).

Changes in population size and structure also affect the demand and supply of various regional public services and the housing market. The declining population can stagnate the real estate (especially, housing) market due to the decline in housing demand over the long term (Sung, 2013). It is difficult to maintain public facilities and infrastructure as demand for urban facilities declines. Then, public facilities and infrastructure will be outdated, and living facilities will be difficult to provide.

The problem is that if the quantity and quality of public services deteriorate due to the declining population and the aging population, a vicious cycle may occur, which accelerates the population outflow. The economic growth rate slowed down by the aging of the population leads to a decline in jobs and income, which in turn leads to a decline in tax revenue, which in turn deteriorates public infrastructure and living conditions. In this case, if a younger population is drained to other regions for jobs or better living conditions, a vicious cycle will occur in which the aging of the region accelerates (Ells, 2008). In this way, if basic public services cannot be provided smoothly due to the declining population and the aging population, the local vitality will fall and local regions can be hollowed out (Wiechmann & Pallagst, 2012). This is the risk of population decline and aging.

As a result, low fertility and aging can be a serious burden on South Korean (hereafter, Korean) society by slowing down economic growth and increasing welfare demand (Ko & Huh, 2015). Population aging and decline of the working age population decrease the vitality of the economy and increase the burden of welfare, which can have a negative impact on economic growth and finance (Yoon & Han, 2018). Korea has experienced a 'Demographic Bonus' period that has experienced economic growth with the growing proportion of the working age population. However, from the time when the productive population decreases, Korea will now face a 'Demographic Onus' period in that consumption and production are at the same time shrinking, and the number of elderly people who need to be supported will increase and the economic growth will slow down (Je & Lee, 2017).

4.3 Population Problems of Local Government in Korea

The problem of population decline and aging of Korean society may be even more serious at the local level. In a region where population aging is relatively rapid, the outflow of the youth population is likely to accelerate the pace of aging. As a result, population aging can be more serious in these areas. In other words, unlike the whole country, population aging, declining population and decreasing economic activity can cause a vicious cycle that deepens mutual negative effects due to interregional population movements. Therefore, if population aging is different in each region, balanced regional development will become difficult, and regional hollowing-out or regional polarization may deepen.

In Japan, where population aging is ahead of us, relative population aging and population decline have accelerated in regions with a low population, resulting in regional integration. Though 75% of Japanese municipalities are declining in population, population decline are accelerating in less populated areas. The metropolis also has a declining population, but its speed is slower than in other regions. Thus, the population concentration towards the metropolis is relatively higher. As a result, population problems at the local level may be more serious, as the impact of aging varies by region. (Yoon & Han, 2018).

In fact, in the case of Korea, the problem of population decline and demographic change is considered serious at the local level (Kim, 2016). In recent years, the problem of the declining population and aging population at the local level is so serious that the term 'local extinction' becomes an issue. The term 'local extinction' expresses a prediction for Japanese society in that the population decline and the pace of aging differ from region to region and only the big cities will survive. Hiroshi Masuda (2015) used 'the proportion of fertile women (20–39 years old)' in the area as an indicator of the possibility of local extinction, because if the female population of these ages does not stay in the area, that area would be difficult to maintain.

After analyzing Korea using the same method, it is expected that 84.1% of the country's 82 counties will disappear within 30 years (Lee, 2016a). In addition, one study used the 16 indicators of population, industry, and physical environment etc. to calculate 'the combined decline index' of the areas (Lee, Oh, & Lee, 2012). The analysis also showed that the level of decline of the population and the aging population are very serious.

Population decline and aging can have a negative impact on local communities, which stagnates the local economy and the real estate market, and reduces public goods' demand. The demand for welfare also increases. This process can deteriorate community well-being. The mechanisms by which population decline and aging deteriorate community well-being, are as follows.

First, if the local economy is stagnated due to the population decline, major industries within the region will be reduced, withdrawn, or transferred. This can lead to a vicious cycle of population decline by increasing the unemployed, and reducing tax revenue and job opportunities. Second, population decline and aging reduce the demand of local public goods. Reducing the overall demand for public goods

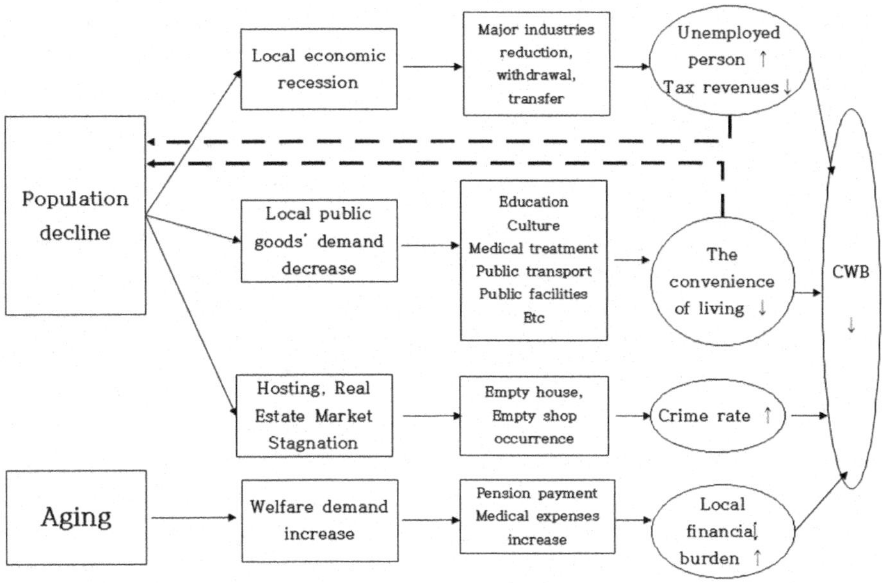

Fig. 4.1 The mechanism by which population decline and aging affect community well-being

such as education, culture, medical care, and public transportation makes it difficult to maintain public infrastructure necessary for public facilities and physical city operation, thus reducing the convenience of residents. This again spills the younger generation population, which can also cause a vicious cycle of population decline. Next, population decline and aging will stagnate the real estate market. When housing demand and development demand decrease, vacant houses and vacant stores are generated, which deteriorates the housing environment by increasing the crime rate. In addition, aging increases pension payments and medical expenses, which increases welfare costs and burdens local finance.

Through this process, population decline and aging will result in a vicious cycle that lowers the well-being of the local community, which in turn reduces the population and accelerates the aging (Fig. 4.1).

Restructured with reference to studies such as Won, Chae, and Song (2010) and Je (2018).

4.4 Korea's Local Government and Migration Intention of Residents

Local governments in Korea are not only facing natural population declines due to low birth rates, but also social population decrement resulting from the outflow of populations to other regions. In Korea, population concentration is clearly in some metropolitan areas. To many local governments, population reduction resulting from the outflow of residents to other regions is a matter of survival and independence (Lee, 2018).

As we have seen, the declining population can accelerate aging and deteriorate conditions of the community, leading to a decline in population. Thus, the decline in population at the local level is a serious problem as it can intensify regional hollowing-out and polarization. Therefore, local governments are attempting to cope with various policy measures to solve the problem of population decline and aging. Population policy at the local level is largely expressed in terms of 'giving birth', 'taking', 'searching', and 'keeping' the population (Lee, 2016b). Some of the typical policies include providing incentives for childbirth, supporting retirees' migration to rural areas, supporting the transfer of resident registration as well as policies that can attract business and create jobs.

However, the policy of 'keeping' the residents in terms of local government can be relatively realistic and effective. It may be easier to prevent the outflow of existing local residents rather than raise the fertility rate and infuse the population from other regions. Because residence transfers involve costs, it is highly likely that local residents will not migrate unless the benefit of the migration exceeds the cost.

In this respect, the policy of 'keeping' local people is important to the local government. Therefore, 'continuing migration intention', which means the degree of intention of residents to continue to live in the present area, is an important concern. Migration intention may be an indicator of the satisfaction and assessment of the residents' current local government services and may be a condition that should be considered in the formulation of local government policy plans in the future. Therefore, despite the fact that actual migration and migration intention do not necessarily coincide, persistent migration intention of residents is important information in itself.

The purpose of this study is to analyze the factors influencing the persistent migration intention of residents and to identify the influence of community well-being on the migration intention in the Korean context. This is because if the policy to raise the level of community well-being increases the willingness to live, it will be a way to confirm that it can be a key solution to the local population problem. In Sect. 4.5, we look at the continuing migration intention.

4.5 Migration Intention of Residents

Migration intention refers to resident's intention to continue to live in a present region. Migration intention could be an important variable to local governments that feel a sense of crisis of sustainability of the local area. Korea is having a problem of low birthrate and aging, and most local governments are feeling the problem of population decline except for some metropolitan areas and a limited number of cities. Population decline of local regions can cause the decrease of local taxes, local finances, and local administrative organizations, which as a result can deteriorate the level of quality and quantity of local services. This also leads to a vicious circle

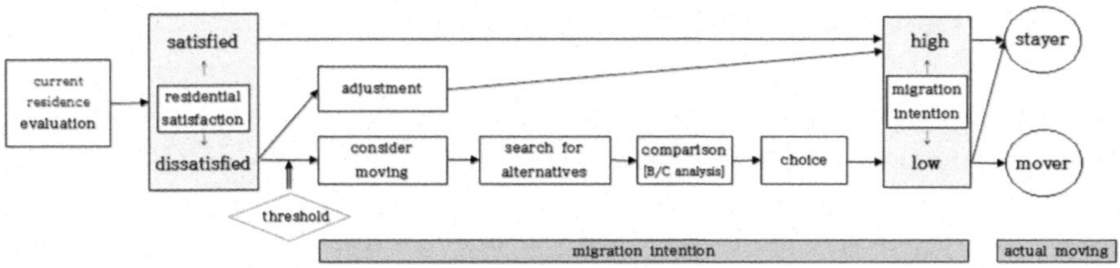

Fig. 4.2 Decision-making process of migration intentions

of resident exit, and generates local hollowization and regional polarization (Lee, 2016b; Yoon & Han, 2018). Hence, local governments try to maintain and increase the population within the region, and resident's migration intention is the concern of local government.

The process of making a migration decision is examined in previous studies (Rossi, 1955; Speare, 1974; Wolpert, 1965). Residents evaluate their current community and neighbors, and then are satisfied or dissatisfied about the current residence on the basis of their evaluation. If the resident's dissatisfaction about the current community exceeds the threshold, they try to adjust to the present region, or consider to move to another area. If the residents consider to migrate, they research other regions to migrate to, compare the alternatives with current regions, and then they decide to move. If there are no satisfactory alternatives, the residents decide to stay in the current residence. This can be expressed as follows (Fig. 4.2).

4.5.1 Lee and Lee (Work-in-Progress)

Through the decision-making process of migration above, we can confirm some of the following. First, 'residential satisfaction' is a crucial factor affecting migration intention. If the level of satisfaction with the current residence is high, the willingness to live is high, but if the level of dissatisfaction exceeds the threshold, people start to consider migration. Second, migration intention is different from actual migration. The consideration of migration does not usually lead to migration (Speare, 1974). Even if migration is considered, migration does not occur if the appropriate alternative area is not found. Or if there is no advantage in comparison with the present area, migration does not occur. On the other hand, even if there is willingness to live in this area, they often migrate by personal/household factors such as a work shift or divorce (Speare, 1974).

Therefore, residential satisfaction alone does not determine the actual move or the decision to move. Nevertheless, prior studies have shown that migration intentions generally reflect behavior and patterns of actual migration (Lansing & Mueller, 1967; Speare, 1974; Von Reichert, 2006). Therefore, previous studies have emphasized migration intention as an important variable in migration studies.

4.6 The Determinants of Migration Intentions

As we have seen, 'residential satisfaction' is a decisive factor for the residents' migration intention. The 'residential satisfaction model' of Speare (1974) is one of the major models of migration research and is a representative initial study (Oh, 2003). Speare (1974) found that most of the background factors (e.g., age and income) have an indirect influence on migration intention through 'residential satisfaction'. Speare distinguished the determinants of migration intention as the factors of background and residential satisfaction. Background factors are also again divided into personal/household factors, local factors, and social bonds with other people (friends and relatives).

Other preceding studies include the following. Oh (2003) divides residential factors into individual/household characteristics, regional characteristics, and again regional characteristics into social bonds and other characteristics based on Speare's model (1974). Heaton, Fredrickson, Fuguitt, and Zuiches (1979) divides economic and non-economic factors (satisfaction, evaluation and preference) into two categories. Von Reichert (2006) divides individual, regional and psychological characteristics.

However, the determinants of migration intention can be basically divided into individual/household, social relation and community factors. Considering the preceding study, this study suggests the following determinants and classification structure of migration intention (Table 4.1).

First, the influence factors of residents can be divided into three major aspects: individual/household characteristics, social relation characteristics, and local community characteristics. Individual/household characteristics can be subdivided into life cycle factors (age, marital status and household size), objective socioeconomic characteristics (household income and educational attainment, employment status) and other factors (gender, home ownership and duration of residence).

Previous studies have shown that age, home ownership, and duration of residence among individual/household characteristics have a significant impact on migration intention. As age, income and seniority privileges increase, satisfaction of residence by itself can increase. In addition, migration intention increases as the satisfaction of the residence increases through the same way as purchasing a satisfactory house (Speare, 1974).

McGinnis (1968) describes the reduction in the probability of moving as the time of residence increase as the axiom of 'the cumulative inertia'. Speare (1974) explains that the longer the residence time, the easier it is for social bonds to be formed. More friends and more familiarity with the use of local facilities and services, the higher the satisfaction of residence. An increase in residential satisfaction also increases the migration intention.

Home ownership is also a very significant factor in increasing migration intention. This is interpreted because people who own their home are motivated to improve the community, and thus, they invest in local amenities and social capital (Rohe & Stewart, 1996). Those who own their homes have the opportunity to become involved

Table 4.1 The determinants of migration intentions

Component		Variables	Previous studies
Individual or household	Life cycle	Age[a]	Kan and Kim (1981), Speare (1974), Von Reichert (2006)
		Marital status	Kan an Kim (1981), Oh (2003)
		Household size	Kan and Kim (1981)
	Objective SES	Household income	Kan and Kim (1981), Oh (2003), Ulrich-Schad et al. (2013)
		Education	Kan and Kim (1981), Speare et al. (1982), Ulrich-Schad et al. (2013)
		Employment status	Kan and Kim (1981), Oh (2003)
	Other	Gender	Oh (2003), Ulrich-Schad et al. (2013)
		Home ownership[a]	Kan and Kim (1981), Oh (2003) Speare (1974)
		Duration of residence[a]	Kan and Kim (1981), Oh (2003), Speare et al. (1982), Von Reichert (2006)
Social relation	Individual social bonds	Friends & relatives	Kan and Kim (1981), Oh (2003), Speare (1974)
	Community social bonds[a]	• Trust • Participation • Cohesion • Attachment	Oh (2003), Speare et al. (1982), Ulrich-Schad et al. (2013)
Community	Objective condition	Community size & density	Von Reichert (2006)
		Community Economic structure	Ulrich Schad et al. (2013), Von Reichert (2006)
	Attitude (psychology)	Community Evaluation • Satisfaction[a]	Kan and Kim (1981), Oh (2003), Speare (1974), Speare et al. (1982), Ulrich-Schad et al. (2013), Von Reichert (2006)

[a]*Note* The asterisk indicates that previous research has been found to be a very strong determinant of migration intention

in organized community organizations in order to protect their interests, to become acquainted with their neighbors, and to feel stronger community bonds and common sense. Thus, they want to live longer in the present area (Lansing & Mueller, 1967).

The characteristics of social relations can be divided into individual dimension and local dimension. First, the presence of friends and relatives in the community influence residents' intentions, which implies the social bonds at the individual level, and has been shown to influence the adaptation and satisfaction of the community (Kan & Kim, 1981; Speare, 1974).

The social dimension of social relations means the social bonds at the local level, and is expressed as 'trust in local community and local neighborhood', 'community activities and participation', and 'attachment and belonging'. The higher the social ties, the higher the migration intention (Oh, 2003; Speare, 1974). The term of social bonds, which is often used in the study of migration intention, means community capital in a general sense.

Community characteristics, one of the determinants of migration intention, can be divided into objective condition and psychological attitude. First, in terms of objective conditions of community, region size, population density, economic structure and conditions have an influence on migration intention. In terms of psychological attitude toward the community, the evaluation and satisfaction of the community affect the migration intention.

The distinction between rural and urban reveals the difference in the objective conditions of the community. In fact, the analysis shows that there is a difference in the migration intention of residents in rural and urban areas. In rural and less populated areas far from a metropolitan area, the population has been seen to hollow out because of the relatively low migration intention (Ulrich-Schad, Henly, & Safford, 2013).

The psychological attitude toward the community is analyzed as a very important determinant of migration intention. The evaluation and satisfaction of the community were analyzed to have a large and consistent effect on the migration intention (Kan & Kim, 1981; Oh, 2003; Speare, 1974; Speare, Kobrin, & Kingkade, 1982; Ulrich-Schad et al., 2013; Von Reichert, 2006).

4.7 Analysis of Determinants of Migration Intention in the Korean Context

4.7.1 Data and Characteristics of the Sample

The data is the "2017 Community Well-being National Survey". It is a survey conducted by the Community Well-being Research Center to measure the level of community well-being of Korea and to seek policy guides for community well-being. The core of the survey is 37 questions about the evaluation of the community and the individual satisfaction of the residents. The survey also includes a number of questions related to life satisfaction and quality of life.

The samples were extracted by the proportion of population by gender and age after forced allocation by 100 persons over some regions. The survey was conducted by a face-to-face interview survey using structured questionnaires from October to November 2017. Among 2,700 valid samples, 2,611 samples excluding 89 with no responses were analyzed in this study. Demographic characteristics of respondents were as follows (Table 4.2).

Table 4.2 Demographic characteristics of the sample

Variables	Educational attainment	Frequency (person)	Proportion (%)	Variables	Social status		Frequency (person)	Proportion (%)
Level	Less than elementary school	202	7.5	Gender	Male		1,339	49.6
	Middle School	292	10.9		Female		1,361	50.4
	High school	1,144	42.5	Marital status	Single		522	19.4
	College or university	1,011	37.6		Married		2,063	76.6
	Above graduate school	40	1.5		Divorce Separation Bereavement		109	4.1
	No answer	11	0.4		No answer		6	0.2
Household income	Less than 1 million won	108	4.0	Religion	Religion	Buddhism	347	12.9
	Over 1 million won ~ less than 2 million won	317	11.8			Protestant	465	17.2
	Over 2 million won ~ less than 3 million won	441	16.4			Catholic	146	5.4
	Over 3 million won ~ less than 4 million won	625	23.2			Other	2	0.1
	Over 4 million ~ less than 5 million won	540	20.1		No religion		1,740	64.4
	Over 5 million won ~ less than 6 million won	394	14.7		N = 2,700			
	Over 6 million won	264	9.8					
	No answer	11	0.4					

4.8 Research Framework and Research Methodology

The purpose of this study is to examine what factors are the determinants of migration intention in the Korean context. In addition to the determinants of previous research, this study attempts to analyze whether the recognition of socioeconomic status (SES) within the region affects migration intention. Since Korea is a society with strong competition and individualism, the perception of the social status on oneself can have a significant effect on the behavior, perception, and intention of the individual. In previous studies, subjective SES perception was found to affect satisfaction and happiness. Therefore, in this study, we will analyze the effect of subjective SES as an individual aspect of social relations on migration intention. This is because the influences of social relations on migration intention may be different from other countries in the Korean context (Fig. 4.3).

Social capital and social solidarity at the collective level have also been identified as major influencing factors for migration intention in prior studies (Speare et al., 1982). The higher the level of trust and bond with the community, or the more experienced in the community, the higher the migration intention. However, the case of Korea may be different.

During the past six decades, Korea has been undergoing rapid industrialization and urbanization, with the rural community becoming stagnant and disintegrating, and the urban community underdeveloped (Lee, 2006). Therefore, it is a general evaluation that local communities have not actively formed in Korea. In this respect, the influence of social capital on individual's intention and behavior may not be large.

On the contrary, as competition intensifies and the individualism tendency is strengthened (Lee, 2006), perceptions and evaluation of self-status in social relations, that is, subjective SES, can act as a factor of migration intention. In this study, multiple regression analysis is performed by adding subjective SES recognition

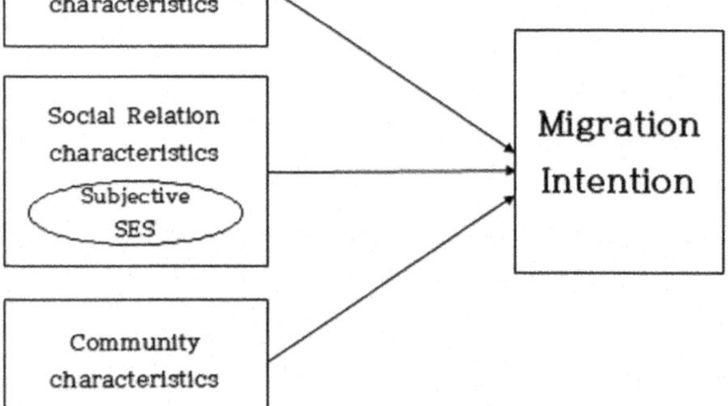

Fig. 4.3 Research framework

variables to existing determinants of migration intention. Since the Breusch-Pagan test showed heteroskedasticity, this study tried to solve this problem by using the heteroskedasticity-robust standard error.

4.9 Measurement of Variables

4.9.1 Dependent Variable: Continuous Migration Intention

Migration intention refers to the degree of resident's intention to continue living in the present community. In this study, migration intention is asked in the following items: "What do you think about continuing to live in the current region? The response consists of a scale of 1 (very low) to 10 (very high), which means that the higher the score, the higher the willingness to continue to live in the present community.

4.9.2 Independent Variables 1: Individual/Household Characteristics

This study considers age, marital status, gender, household size, household income, educational attainment, employment status, home ownership, and duration of residence as individual/household characteristics. The dummy variables were gender (male = 0, female = 1), economic activity (inactivity = 0, activity = 1), and ownership status (self-ownership = 0, ownership = 1). Other variables were measured as follows: age as full age; marital status as (1) unmarried, (2) married, (3) divorced, or (4) separated; educational attainment as (1) elementary school, (2) middle school, (3) high school, (4) college and university, and (5) graduate school or higher.

4.9.3 Independent Variable 2: Social Relation Characteristics

This study deals with two aspects of social relations of the community: social capital (trust, network, and bonds) as the collective aspect and 'subjective SES' recognition as the individual aspect. In this study, however, we could not deal with the aspect of personal and social 'friends or relatives' because of the limitation of data. First, we focus on trust, network, and social bonds at the local level as subordinate components of social capital. The core elements of social capital can be seen as networks and trust, because these two factors have been emphasized in many previous studies, and individuals' attitudes toward social 'networks' appear through 'trust'. In addition to the two elements, this study includes 'social bonds' as a component. This is because social bonds have a cognitive attribute that is different from trust and is emphasized in previous studies. Trust is a belief in reciprocity in the exchange of resources (Lee, 2009). The network means that individuals have a linkage structure within a society. Social bonds also refer to the sense of solidarity and unity felt in the network and its members.

The specific measurements are as follows. Trust was measured as "how satisfied are you with the trust of the local residents or local government?" The network was measured as "how satisfied are you with the participation of community organizations?" Social bonds were measured as 'how satisfied are you with your community's tenacity and cooperation activities?' Since network in itself is difficult to measure, the study has measured the participation and activities within the network structure.

The responses of each question consisted of a 10-point scale (1 = highly dissatisfied ~ 10 = very satisfied), and local social capital was measured as the sum of trust, network, bond and each item. Social capital is an intangible resource inherent in the structure of relationships among actors and is not as readily measurable as traditional capital. For this reason, previous studies measured social capital as a phenomenon perceived by individuals (Koo & Park, 2015). Although measuring social capital as 'perceived social capital' may differ from objectively existing social capital, researching perceived social capital is a meaningful alternative because the social capital must undergo a 'cognitive process' before it can affect an individual's behavior.

The subjective socioeconomic status was also measured by the following items: "What is your socioeconomic status in your community? Please tell me the number between the phases of ① the lowest class ~ ⑨ the highest class". In other words, the response consists of a 9-point scale, and the higher the response value, the higher the socioeconomic status within the region.

4.9.4 Independent Variable 3: Community Characteristics

This study reflected community characteristics as residential satisfaction and rural-urban division variables. Residential satisfaction was measured as the sum of satisfaction with a total of 28 questions about local conditions and states (e.g., library, public transport, and jobs). The results of the confirmatory factor analysis of 28 items measuring residential satisfaction showed that the factor loadings of all the measurement items were 0.50 or more, statistically significant, and Cronbach's value of 0.96. The response is on a 10-point scale (1 = very unsatisfied ~ 10 = very satisfied) and the higher the response value, the higher the local satisfaction.

In addition, the urban and rural areas are generally classified according to local population size, rurality, and economic dependency (Ulrich-Schad et al., 2013; Von Reichert, 2006). This study classified urban and rural areas according to the classification table of the local governments of the directive of the Ministry of Government Administration and Home Affairs: ① large city type; ② small and medium city type; ③ limited urban type; ④ rural and city mixed type; and ⑤ rural type. In this study, the rural, and rural and urban mixed type was classified into rural type and the rest was classified into urban/city type (0 = rural type, 1 = urban type).

4.10 Analysis Results

The results of the analysis of the determinants of migration intention are shown in Table 4.3.

The results showed that marital status, household income, educational attainment, employment status, and gender affect migration intention among the individual/household factors. Also, a married and employed person showed higher migration intention. In addition, the higher the household income, the higher the migration intention. The results of this study are different from the previous studies in that the higher the household income, the higher the residents' intention to live in the present community. In Korea, it seems that households with a lot of income move to better residential areas, because buying a house in good condition is used as a means of proliferating assets.

However, the larger the household size, the higher the attainment of education, the lower the migration intention. Women showed lower migration intentions than men, and these results are generally consistent with previous studies. On the other hand, analysis shows that age, homeownership, and duration of residence do not significantly affect migration intention. This is remarkable in that it is a very different result from the previous study. In general, this can be interpreted as a result of Korea's

Table 4.3 The results of analysis

Variables		Beta	Robust S.E.
Individual or household	Age	−0.02	0.00
	Marital status	0.07***	0.08
	Household size	−0.04*	0.03
	Household income	0.05**	0.02
	Educational attainment	−0.07**	0.04
	Employment status dummy	0.01	0.06
	Gender dummy	−0.03*	0.05
	Home ownership dummy	0.01	0.06
	Duration of residence	0.00	0.00
Social relation	Subjective SES	0.07***	0.03
	Social capital	0.11***	0.04
Community	Rural city dummy	−0.15***	0.05
	Community well-being	0.41***	0.00
Observations		2611	
F(df)		(13,2597)49.21	
R^2		0.26	
vif		1.89	

* Significant at 0.1 level, ** Significant at 0.05 level, *** Significant at 0.01 level

high mobility in the process of urbanization and industrialization within a short period of time. However, it is necessary to further analyze the reason for this.

Next, social relation characteristics were found to affect migration intention in both collective and individual aspects. The social capital of the region and the individual subjective SES both have a positive (+) influence on migration intention. In other words, the higher the social capital and the higher the subjective SES within the region, the higher the migration intention.

The results of the analysis are noteworthy in that they differ from the general assessment that local communities are underdeveloped. In Korea's rapid industrialization and urbanization, rural communities have been stagnated and urban communities have been underdeveloped. Thus, the influence of social capital at the local level may not be significant. However, the results of the analysis show that the impact of social capital is greater than that of individual subjective SES. This result is noteworthy in that the local capital in Korea affects the migration intention of the individual and may also play an important role in residential satisfaction.

Finally, looking at the characteristics of the community, it was found that both objective condition and subjective perception or satisfaction had a significant effect on migration intention. Urban and rural variables, which indicate the objective characteristics of the region, showed that the urban residents had a low intention to live in the present community. Community well-being, which indicates community satisfaction, has a positive influence on migration intention. In particular, the coefficients of the community well-being variables are very high, indicating that they are very significant and strong resident affecting factors in comparison to other variables.

Overall, community and social factors were found to be important factors in migration intention. In addition, we can confirm that the well-being level of community measured subjective perception and satisfaction of community is a very important factor of migration intention.

4.11 Conclusions

This study started with the recognition that migration intention of local residents could be a major concern for local governments in Korea, which suffered not only from declining natural population but also from declining social populations (outflows). Despite the need for research, there is a lack of domestic studies on migration intention. Thus, this study attempts to identify the determinants of migration intention in the Korean context. The main purpose of this study is to confirm whether or not the residents' perception of community well-being affects migration intention.

As a result of the analysis, it was confirmed that there is a need to further analyze the difference of characteristics between Korea and other countries, because the individual/household characteristics are slightly different from those of studies abroad. For example, there is a need to explore why age, home ownership and duration of residence, which are highly emphasized in studies abroad, do not have a significant impact on migration intention.

Second, the characteristics of social relations at the local level have a significant effect on the migration intention of residents. Above all, it is noteworthy that the social capital of the region has a significant influence on the migration intention of the residents, despite the evaluation of the lack of growth and development of the local community as a result of rapid urbanization and industrialization in Korea. It has been confirmed that local trust, social bonds, and participation in community organizations can be important to the migration intention of residents. In addition, we analyzed the subjective SES within the region, which were not noticed in previous studies, and confirmed the significant effect on migration intention.

Finally, the influence of community characteristics on migration intention was confirmed. This study tried to analyze the objective characteristics of the community through the distinction between urban and rural areas with different population sizes, structure, and economic characteristics. As a result, the objective characteristics of the community affected the migration intentions.

However, it is noteworthy that residents' awareness of community well-being has a great influence on migration intention. As a result, increasing the level of community well-being for local governments experiencing population decline is not only the method to improve the quality of life and satisfaction of local residents, but also an alternative to maintaining the population by increasing the migration intention of local residents. And promoting community well-being is the way to maintain and develop the area. That is why local governments should be more interested in community well-being.

Acknowledgements This work was supported by the National Research Foundation of Korea Grant funded by the Korean Government (NRF-2016S1A3A2924563).

References

Elis, V. (2008). The impact of the ageing society on regional economies. In *The demographic challenge: A handbook about Japan* (pp. 861–878).

Heaton, T., Fredrickson, C., Fuguitt, G. V., & Zuiches, J. J. (1979). Residential preferences, community satisfaction, and the intention to move. *Demography, 16*(4), 565–573.

Hiroshi, M. (2015). *Local decay* (J.-H. Kim, Trans.). Wiseberry.

Je, H. J., & Lee, H. Y. (2017). Regional demographic change and characteristic analysis by type. *Korean Journal of Urban Geography, 20*(1), 27–43.

Je, H. J. (2018). *Actual conditional of classified types of regional population decrease and the comparison of urban planning responses*. Ph.D. thesis, Seoul National University.

Kan, S. H., & Kim, Y. (1981). Religious affiliation and migration intentions in nonmetropolitan Utah. *Rural Sociology, 46*(4), 669.

Kim, S. E. (2016). National and regional responses to low fertility and aging society and population decline. In *2016 Korea-Japan Joint Seminar, 30 November, 2016*.

Ko, Y. H., & Huh, J. W. (2015). The age of population decline, over development problems and policy direction. *Korea Regional Economics Research, 33,* 87–103.

Koo, Y. Y., & Park, I. K. (2015). The relationship between immigrant social capital and community adaptation. *Urban Administration, 28*(4), 53–76.

Lansing, J., & Mueller, E. (1967). *The geographic mobility of labor*. Ann Arbor: Institute of Social Research.

Lee, J. K. (2009). Satisfaction with life and social capital: Centered on the effect of civic participation, trust and social resources. *Studies in Humanities and Social Sciences, 22,* 5–40.

Lee, J. Y. (2006). Community and social capital. Korea Society of Social Sciences Symposium, 23–49.

Lee, S. H. (2016a). *Seven analysis on the local extinction in Korea, regional employment trend brief.* Korea Employment Information Service.

Lee, S. Y. (2016b). Rehabilitation plan of local government in response to local disappearance. *Urban Problems, 51*(577), 24–27.

Lee, S. Y., Oh, E. J., & Lee, H. Y. (2012*). Regional decline analysis and regression analysis*. Korea Institute of Local Government Administration.

Lee, Y. K. (2018). The relationship between local governments' policy orientation and population movement: Exploring the possibility of local governments' redistribution policy. *Journal of Korean Public Administration, 52*(2), 301–335.

McGinnis, R. (1968). A stochastic model of social mobility. *American Sociological Review,* 712–722.

Oh, J.-H. (2003). Social bonds and the migration intentions of elderly urban residents: The mediating effect of residential satisfaction. *Population Research and Policy Review, 22*(2), 127–146.

Rohe, W. M., & Stewart, L. S. (1996). Homeownership and neighborhood stability. *Housing Policy Debate, 7*(1), 37–81.

Rossi, P. H. (1955). *Why families move: A study in the social psychology of urban residential mobility*. Free Press.

Speare, A. (1974). Residential satisfaction as an intervening variable in residential mobility. *Demography, 11*(2), 173–188.

Speare, A., Jr., Kobrin, F., & Kingkade, W. (1982). The influence of socioeconomic bonds and satisfaction on interstate migration. *Social Forces, 61*(2), 551–574.

Statistics Korea. (2016). Future population estimate, 2015–2065.

Sung, Y. D. (2013). A study on the demographic change and housing policy in Korea. *Real Estate Journal, 53,* 224–237.

Ulrich-Schad, J. D., Henly, M., & Safford, T. G. (2013). The role of community assessments, place, and the great recession in the migration intentions of rural Americans. *Rural Sociology, 78*(3), 371–398.

Von Reichert, C. (2006). Community evaluation and migration intentions. In *Population change and rural society* (pp. 333–356). Springer.

Wiechmann, T., & Pallagst, K. M. (2012). Urban shrinkage in Germany and the USA: A comparison of transformation patterns and local strategies. *International Journal of Urban and Regional Research, 36*(2), 261–280.

Wolpert, J. (1965). Behavioral aspects of the decision to migrate. *Papers in Regional Science, 15*(1), 159–169.

Won, K. H., Chae, S. J., & Song, C. S. (2010). *Strategies to revitalizing shrinking cities in a population-declining era: Through the small- and medium-sized cities of Korea*. Chungbuk Research Institute.

Yoon, S. H., & Han, S. W. (2018). Possible reduction of productionable population and potential for local autonomous entrenchment. KRI report issue analysis (pp. 18–21).

YeonKyeong Lee is a research fellow at the Center for Well-being Research at the Korean Institute of Public Affairs, Seoul National University, South Korea. In August 2017, she received a Ph.D. in public policy from the Graduate School of Public Administration, Seoul National University. The doctoral dissertation is "The study on the relationship between policy orientation of local governments and migration". Major areas of interest are local government's behavior and policy, residents' happiness, welfare policy and local finance.

Seung Jong Lee is a Professor and Dean of the Graduate School of Public Administration, Seoul National University. Previously, he served as the president of the Korean Association for Public Administration and as chief editor of several academic journals in related fields. He has frequently advised local and national governments through such positions as chairman of the Local Government Administration Joint Evaluation Committee, vice-chairman of the Presidential Committee on Local District Reorganization Plans, and member of the presidential transition committee. He has not only done extensive research on citizen participation and local autonomy but has also been a strong advocate and educator in the field. He is the author of *Theories of Local Autonomy*, and *Democratic Politics and Citizen Participation*.

Chapter 5
Perceived Social Support Systems for Bereaved Students in Walter Sisulu University: A Pilot Study

Sabi Baninzi and T. Mdleleni-Bookholane

Abstract The purpose of this study was to examine perceived social support systems for bereaved students in institutions of higher learning with specific reference to Walter Sisulu University (WSU). One hundred and eighty-two (182) first year students who were between ages 15 and 36 years and above with the mean age of 25.5 were selected from three faculties. The data were collected using a questionnaire and a Multidimensional Scale of Perceived Social Support (MSPSS) by Zimet et al. (J Pers Assess 52:30–41, 1988). The themes for the questionnaire included prevalence of bereavement, help-seeking behavioral patterns in relation to gender, and ways of improving the quality of life for grieving students. The Multidimensional Scale of Perceived Social Support (MSPSS) assessed three sources of support available to students (e.g., family (FA), friends (FR), and significant other (SO). Data collected was analyzed using SPSS. Findings showed that a significant number of students had suffered more than one loss of someone close to them through death in the past 24 months; most students got social support from either family, friends, person or community members who were willing to help; majority of female students did not know of any place on campus where they would go to and seek help when they grieve as compared to the male counterparts; and sadly, that some students did not receive any form of assistance on campus when they were grieving.

Keywords Student bereavement · Help-seeking behavior · Social support network · Sources of support

---

S. Baninzi (✉) · T. Mdleleni-Bookholane
Faculty of Humanities, Social Sciences and Law, Department of Social Work and Psychology, Walter Sisulu University, Nelson Mandela Drive, Private Bag X1, Mthatha 5117, Eastern Cape, South Africa
e-mail: sabibaninzi@gmail.com

T. Mdleleni-Bookholane
e-mail: tem.mdleleni@gmail.com

© Springer Nature Switzerland AG 2019

Y. Kee et al. (eds.), *Perspectives on Community Well-Being*, Community Quality-of-Life and Well-Being, https://doi.org/10.1007/978-3-030-15115-7_5

5.1 Introduction

The purpose of the present study was to examine the perceptions of students at WSU regarding social support systems for the bereaved students. Kail and Cavanaugh (2007) define bereavement as a state or condition caused by the loss through death. Grief as the sorrow, hurt, anger, guilt, confusion, and other feelings that arise after suffering a loss. Given high death rates in South Africa, which range from HIV/AIDS-related deaths (AIDS Foundation of South Africa, 2005; Center for Disease Control and Prevention, 2006; Department of Health (DOH), South Africa, 2006; World Bank, 2005; World Health Organization (WHO), 2006), fatal roads accidents (Department of Transport (DOT), South Africa, 2006; UNAIDS, 2006), as well as violent killings, bereavement research is important, but has remained largely under-researched (Somhlaba, 2006). The psychological experience of grieving in South Africa, as well as the role of supportive networks in dealing with bereavement, has remained largely ignored (Spangenberg & Somhlaba, 2003).

The research reported in the present paper was inspired by the work of David Fajgenbaum (2007) who investigated university student bereavement in particular looking at university responses, programs and policies, and recommendations for improvement. Life for university students can be a very difficult consignment and without proper guidance and support this can be detrimental to the students' wellbeing. Servaty-Seib and Taub (2008) have observed that bereavement is a life transition or crisis faced by a significant share of the campus population at any given time. Death, loss experience and subsequent grief reactions have a strong potential to affect the functioning and overall development of bereaved students. Due to the prevalence of university students' bereavement and the widespread inattention to the effects of such losses on young people during this stressful life transition, university students bereavement has been referred to as "silent pandemic" that negatively impacts the bereaved academically, socially, and developmentally (Balk, 2001). Brannon and Feist (2004) argued that failure to acknowledge the problem that can be brought by inability or not dealing with loss of a loved one can have bad consequences to a bereaved student. This can lead to high failure rate, dropouts, physical illness, and most importantly into a mental disorder.

It was against this background that it was important to conduct a study on student bereavement in Walter Sisulu University (WSU). WSU is situated in one of South Africa's poorest province in the Eastern Cape and, as such, is faced with many challenges and problems such as HIV/AIDS pandemic, poverty, unemployment to name a few (AIDS Foundation of South Africa, 2005) (Fig. 5.1).

Most of WSU students come from traditional rural backgrounds, where people were taught not to confide their problems and feelings with strangers. Unresolved bereavement issues coupled with other university stressors can pose a great threat to the bereaved student (Sikkema, Hansen, Meade, Kochman, & Lee, 2005). Brannon and Feist (2004) further highlighted that stress on university students are mainly caused by several factors such as a move from home to university, separation anxiety, and loss of control over a new environment, academic pressures, interpersonal

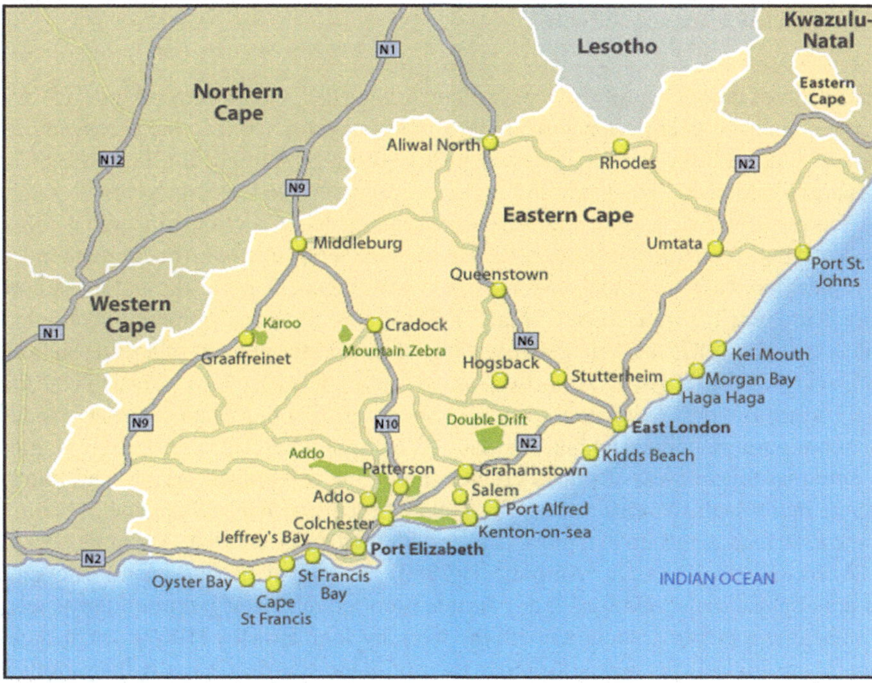

Fig. 5.1 Map showing the Eastern Cape Province of South Africa

problems, financial problems, family problems, social and environmental problems, and homesickness. Furthermore, failure to acknowledge the problem or not dealing with the loss of a loved one can have bad consequences for a bereaved student and this can lead to high failure rates, dropouts, physical illness, and most importantly to mental disorders (Brannon & Feist, 2004). Similarly, Servaty-Seib (2009) state that grief can affect students' academic performance in a number of ways.

Servaty-Seib and Taub (2008) observed that many university students have already experienced a death love one before they come to university. Some experience a death of someone close to them during their university years. If the death of a love one occurs during college years, it can be a more difficult time because the student may be living away from others who are experiencing this same loss and may not know other students well enough to get support that he or she may need (Servaty-Seib & Taub, 2008). This becomes a problem as most of WSU students come from traditional rural background where people were taught not to share their problems and feelings to a stranger. The problem of unresolved bereavement issues coupled with other university stressors can pose great threat to the bereaved student (Sikkema et al., 2005).

5.2 Social Convoy Model

The results of the present study were explained using the Social Convoy Model (SCM) as it recognizes the importance of social support networks to help the bereaved persons to deal with the loss of loved ones. According to Antonucci (2001) the SCM was developed in 1980 by Kahn and Antonucci and modified over the years. It sought to incorporate the developmental and dynamic aspects of relationships into a single model. It builds on the traditionally developmental perspective of Attachment theory, the contextual basis of Role theory, as well as fields of social networks and social support (Antonucci, Birditt, & Akiyama, 2009). According to the extract by Antonucci and Akiyama (1987) the term convoy was first used in the context of social relations by David Plath (1980) in his Anthropological studies of the Japanese. Through the use of the term convoy, Plath meant to convey the notion that individuals are surrounded by a community of others who accompany them throughout their lifetime. He wanted to note that this convoy of others creates something of a protective cocoon, allowing the individuals to move through age-related events with the advantage of being a member of a larger group that moves along with them (Antonucci & Akiyama, 1987).

According to Kahn and Antonucci (1980) the convoys focus on the life-span nature of close social relations. They further reported that SCM incorporated aspects of attachment theory associated with the work by John Bowlby (1969) which states that infants initially become attached to their primary caregiver, usually their mother. The result is a secure attachment that leads to higher levels of competence in children and more successful relationships among adults (Bowlby, 1982). Kahn and Antonucci (1980) also reported that the convoy also incorporates aspects of role theory associated with the work by Mead (1934) and Merton (1957) who described roles as common socially ascribed positions in society, including norms and expectations of behaviour (Kahn & Antonucci, 1980). Whereas attachment theory focuses on individuals, role theory refers to intergroup or societal expectations. Roles might be personal or professional such as being a parent, child, spouse, or factory worker, business executive, politician etc. according to this perspective, multiple roles (e.g., worker, spouse, churchgoer, friend, club member, neighbours) promote greater social connectedness and integration (Moen, 2001). Importantly to note is that roles may be ascribed, developed and achieved through social interaction (Moen, 2001).

The SCM can be viewed as represented as a series of three concentric circles surrounding an individual (Kahn & Antonucci, 1980). This highlights the importance of social support network such as family, friends and significant others in providing social support the bereaved students (see Fig. 5.2).

In trying to explain this further Hough, Magnan, Templin, and Gadelrab (2005) proposed the following steps: firstly, the inclusion of persons in a convoy circle was determined by the individual's emotional attachment to the person as well as by the role of the person in relation to the focal individual (Hough et al., 2005). Secondly, persons occupying the innermost circle of an individual's social convoy were likely to be important support providers with whom the main individual feels very close (Hough et al., 2005). Thirdly, membership in the second circle suggests a degree of

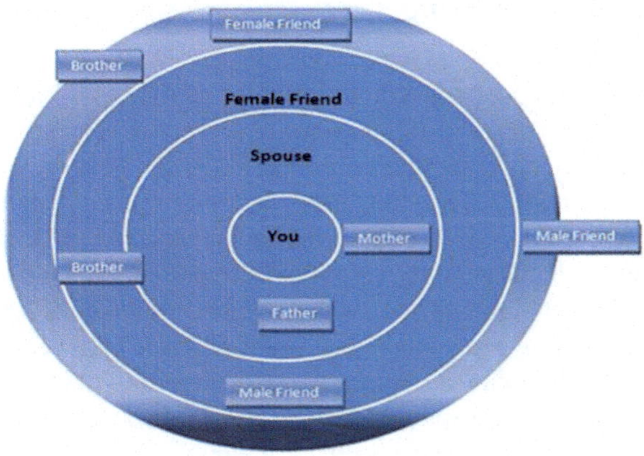

Fig. 5.2 Diagram representing the Social Convoy Model (SCM)

closeness to the focal individual as well as relationships that are based on more than just fulfillment of a role (Hough et al., 2005). Finally, members of the third circle are thought to be close to the focal individual but usually in a very role-prescribed manner. Hough and colleagues further argued that in its entirety, the convoy model evokes an image of a protective layer of family, friends, and others who "surround the individual and help in the successful negotiation of life's challenges" (Antonucci & Akiyama, 1987, p. 516) as the individual moves through life (Hough et al., 2005). Owens (2003) reported that observation in a variety of settings have highlighted the positive roles played by social attachments in psychological adjustment and health. According to Owens these types of observations have led to two ideas that social support offers which are: (a) contributes to positive adjustment and personal development and (b) provides a buffer against the effects of stress (Owens, 2003).

The Social Convoy Model (SCM) is the guiding framework for the present study as the scale (MSPSS) used to collect the data accurately solicited information relating to social support network that is readily available to students, that is the family, friends, and significant others. The SCM also guided the main objective of the study which is to examine social support systems available on campus as perceived by grieving students.

5.3 Research Design and Methods

The study used a Survey research design to gather information from first year students at WSU. The purpose for using this design was that it gives a greater insight into what students perceived to be their social support network when grieving on campus.

5.3.1 Sampling

The study used convenient sampling method to gather 182 participants whom all were in their first year of study at the university. The students were registered for either English for Academic Purposes (EAP) and Communication Skills Program (CSP) in the year 2013. The study used these programs as target population because they were cross-cutting skills offered in English Department done by all first-year students. The rationale of using this group was that they are the ones who are mostly affected by many problems as observed by Brannon and Feist (2004) who emphasized that stress among university students is mainly caused by several factors such as the stress of the transition to university; moves from home to university; separation anxiety and loss of control over the new environment; academic pressures; interpersonal problems; financial problems; family problems; social and environmental problems; loss of someone close and homesickness.

5.3.2 Research Instruments

Two instruments were used to collect data: The questionnaire and Multidimensional Scale of Perceived Social Support (MSPSS) by Zimet, Dahlem, Zimet, and Farley et al. (1988). Both instruments were written in English as all research participants were university students and most importantly doing an English module. The questionnaire covered the following themes: Students' biographical details; the prevalence of bereavement amongst students. The questionnaire consisted of open-ended questions and closed-ended questions which gave the respondents the opportunity to give direct responses and explanations where specified. While the Multidimensional Scale of Perceived Social Support (MSPSS) was used to assess three sources of support available to students (e.g., family (FA), friends (FR), and significant other (SO). The scale was used in its original form and covered the theme on social support systems available as perceived by grieving students.

5.3.3 Pretesting

Reliability and validity of the research instrument was evaluated through piloting which consisted of 12 participants, 6 females and 6 males in order to identify the accuracy and appropriateness of the research instrument (Bless, Smith, & Kagee, 2006).

5.3.4 Procedure for Data Collection

For the data to be collected, permission was obtained from the head of the English Department. After being granted the permission, the researcher arranged with the lecturers concerned regarding the specific class periods so to have an hour to do data collection. Students from both programmes EAP and CSP attended one lecture per week. During that period ethical issues involved in the study were communicated to the students such as voluntary participation, confidentiality and anonymity. The purpose and the importance of conducting the study was also explained. Thereafter, questionnaires were distributed during the lecture period to all students. The researcher was available to students so as to assist the participants by outlining what was needed to be done in answering the questions as well as to help to clarify whatever was not understood in order to ensure that the participants answer all questions correctly. The questionnaires were collected at the end of the lecture, immediately after the students had finished.

5.3.5 Method for Data Analysis

The data were analyzed using a computer software program known as SPSS version 18.0. Then the responses were cross-tabulated to ensure an in-depth interpretation of the results. This program enabled the researcher to have tables that helped the researcher to determine the relationship between variables.

5.4 Results

Table 5.1 shows that there were 182 students that participated, 64 were males and 118 females. Fifty three percent (n-96) were between ages 15 and 20 years, 38.5% (n-70) being females and 14.3% (n-26) males. Forty two percent (n-76) were between ages 21 and 25 years, with 23.1% (n-42) being females and 18.7% (n-34) males. For those who were between ages 26 and 30 years, females were 2.7% (n-5) and 1.6% (n-3) were males. There was only one female who fell in the category of 31–35 years and one male in the category of 36 years and above.

Table 5.2 shows that 93.5% (n-171) were single with 60.5% (n-110) being females and 33.5% (n-61) were males. Three percent (n-3) were married, with 2.2% (n-4) being females and only one male. There was only one female who was in the category of divorced. There was 3% (n-5) of respondents who were cohabiting, with 1.7% (n-3) being females and 1.1% (n-2) were males.

Table 5.3 indicates that majority 69% (n-125) of students were staying on campus residence, that is, 46% (n-84) females and 22% (n-41) males. Of the other 31% (n-57), 19% (n-34) females and 13% (n-23) males were residing outside campus.

Table 5.1 Distribution of students by age and gender

Age and gender	Gender				Total	
	Males		Females			
	Freq	%	Freq	%	Freq	Total (%)
15–20 years	26	14.3	70	38.5	96	53
21–25 years	34	18.7	42	23.1	76	42
26–30 years	3	1.6	5	2.7	8	4.0
31–35 years	0	0	1	0.5	1	0.5
36 years+	1	0.5	0	0	1	0.5
Total	64	35.2	118	64.8	182	100

Table 5.2 Distribution of students by marital status and gender

What is your marital status?	Gender				Total	
	Males		Females			
	Freq	%	Freq	%	Freq	Total (%)
Single	61	33.5	110	60.5	171	93.5
Married	1	0.5	4	2.2	5	3
Divorced	0	0	1	0.5	1	0.5
Cohabiting	2	1.1	3	1.7	5	3
Total	64	35.1	118	64.9	182	100

Table 5.3 Distribution of students by residence and gender

Do you live in residence?	Gender				Total	
	Males		Females			
	Freq	%	Freq	%	Freq	Total (%)
Yes	41	22	84	46	125	69
No	23	13	34	19	57	31
Total	64	35	118	65	182	100

Table 5.4 indicates that 39% (n-71) understood bereavement as "loss of someone close to you," another 31.4% (n-57) understood it as "loss of someone close to you through death". Then 20.3% (N-37) understood bereavement as "unhappy and painful emotion due to loss suffered" while 7.1% (N-13) understood it as "when you lose someone related to you". Only two defined it as "understanding grief and how it affects us" while another two failed to express themselves.

Table 5.4 Students' understanding of bereavement

Bereavement is…	Frequency	Percent	Valid percent	Cumulative percent
Loss of someone close to you through death	57	31.4	31.4	31.4
Loss of someone close to you	71	39.0	39.0	70.4
Lose a person related to you	13	7.1	7.1	77.5
Unhappy and painful emotion due to loss suffered	37	20.3	20.3	97.8
Understanding grief and how it affect us	2	1.1	1.1	98.9
No response	2	1.1	1.1	100.0
Total	182	100.0	100.0	

Table 5.5 Students' number of losses suffered in the past 24 months

Students' number of losses suffered in the past 24 months	Gender				Total	
	Males		Females			
	Freq	%	Freq	%	Freq	Total (%)
1	19	11	40	22	59	33
2	6	3	20	11	26	14
3	8	4	13	7	21	12
4	2	1	7	4	9	5
5	0	–	2	1	2	1
More than 5	2	1	6	3	8	4
None	27	15	30	17	57	31
Total	64	35	118	65	182	100

Table 5.5 shows that majority 33% (n-59) of the students had suffered one loss in the past 24 months, that is, 22% (n-40) females and 11% (n-19) males. While 31% (n-57) had not suffered any loss at all, 17% (n-30) females and 15% (n-27) males. Fourteen percent (N-26) reported suffering two losses that is 11% (n-20) females and 3% (n-6) males, 12% (n-21) reported suffering three losses, 7% (n-13) of females and 4% (n-8) of males. Five percent 5% (N-9) reported suffering four losses that is 4% (n-7) females and 1% (n-2) males. Then 4% (N-8) suffered more than five losses, 3% (n-6) of females and 1% (n-2) of males. Only two female students reported to suffer five losses through death in the past 24 months.

5.4.1 *Social Support Systems Available as Perceived by Grieving Students*

Figure 5.3 illustrates that 4.4% (n-8) very strongly agreed while 36.8% (n-67) strongly agreed and 13.2% (n-24) mildly agreed. Twenty point three percent (n-37) very strongly disagreed while 4.9% (n-9) strongly disagreed and 6.6% (n-12) mildly disagreed. Thirteen point seven percent (n-25) were neutral in their response.

Figure 5.4 demonstrate that 4.4% (n-8) very strongly agreed while 35.7% (n-65) strongly agreed and 25.3% (n-46) mildly agreed with the statement. Thirteen point two percent (n-24) very strongly disagreed while 5.5% (n-10) strongly disagreed and 4.9% (n-9) mildly disagreed. Eleven percent (n-20) were neutral.

Figure 5.5 demonstrates that 5.5% (n-10) very strongly agreed while 51.6% (n-94) strongly agreed and 12.6% (n-23) of them mildly agreed with the statement. Leven point five percent (n-21) very strongly disagreed while 3.8% (n-7) strongly disagreed and 3.3% (n-6) mildly disagreed. Eleven point five percent (n-21) were neutral.

Figure 5.6 shows that 4.9% (n-9) very strongly agreed while 36.3% (n-66) strongly agreed and 16.5% (n-30) mildly agreed with the statement. Ten point four percent (n-19) very strongly disagreed and 8.8% (n-16) strongly disagreed and 6.6% (n-12) mildly disagreed. Sixteen point five percent (n-30) were neutral.

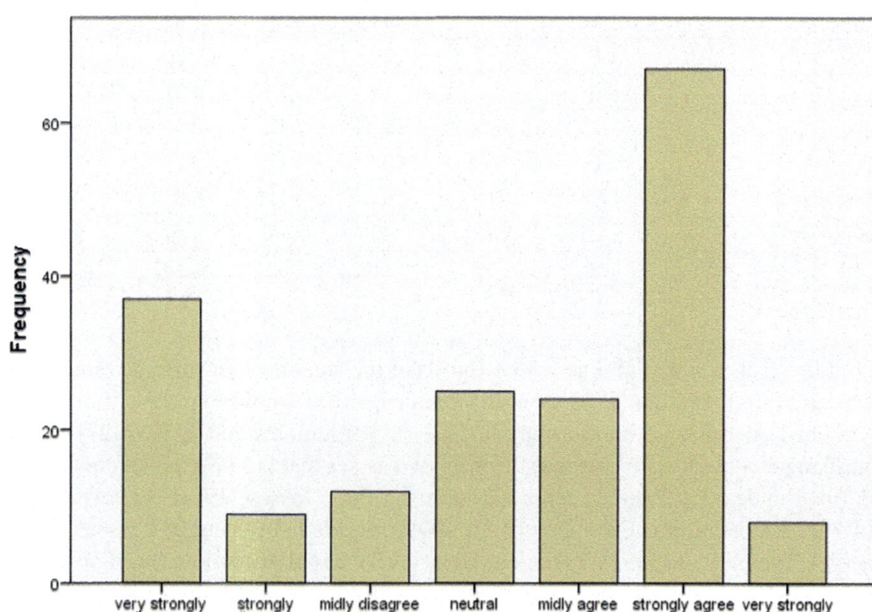

Fig. 5.3 There is a special person who is around when I am in need

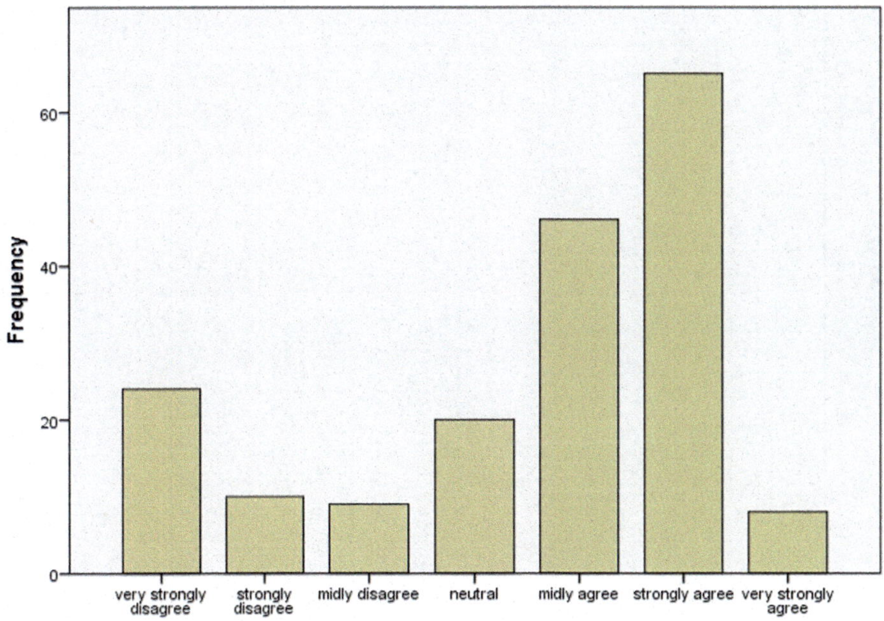

Fig. 5.4 There is a special person with whom I share my joys and sorrows

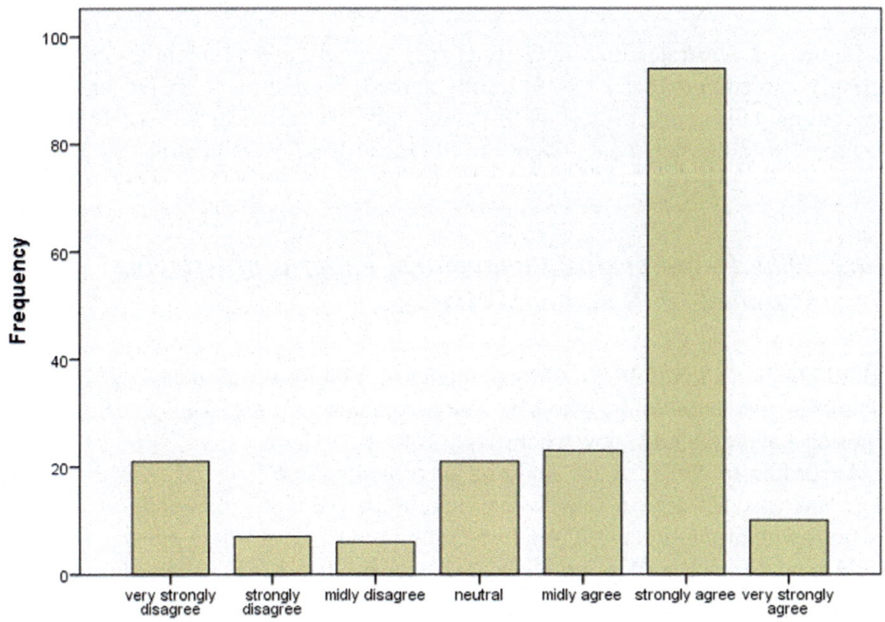

Fig. 5.5 I get the emotional help and support I need from my family

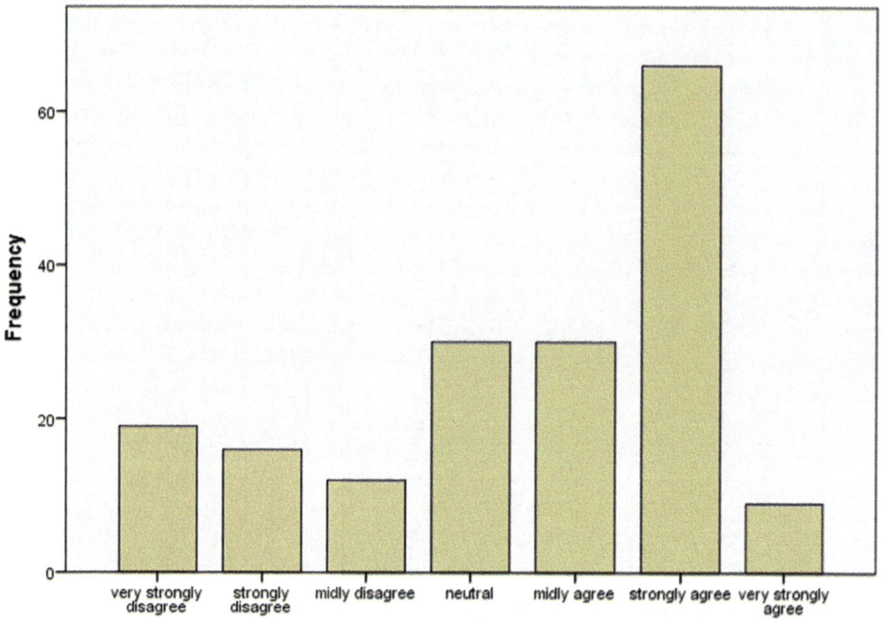

Fig. 5.6 I can talk about my problems with my family

Figure 5.7 illustrates that 4.4% (n-8) very strongly agreed while 29.7% (n-54) strongly agreed and 18.7% (n-34) mildly agreed. Twelve point six percent (n-23) very strongly disagreed while 4.4% (n-8) strongly disagreed and 8.2% (n-15) mildly disagreed with the statement. Twenty two percent (n-40) were neutral.

5.4.2 *The Help-Seeking Behavioural Patterns of Grieving Students in Relation to Gender*

Table 5.6 shows that 82% (n-150) of students, 54% (n-99) females and 28% (n-51) males, would not know where to seek help when grieving. Another 18% (n-32) reported that they would know where to go, 10% (n-19) females and 7% (n-13) males.

According to Table 5.7 the majority of students (56.6%, n-103) suggested that there was a need for free sessions with psychologists, support groups, and counselling sessions with professionals, 32.4% (n-59) suggested a place where grieving students could go and talk about their problems and be given advice (i.e., Counselling Centre) and 8.3% (n-15) did not have any response at all. While 2.2% (n-4) suggested that the university should reopen a Guidance and Counselling Unit (GCU), one student suggested that there should be enough books in the library.

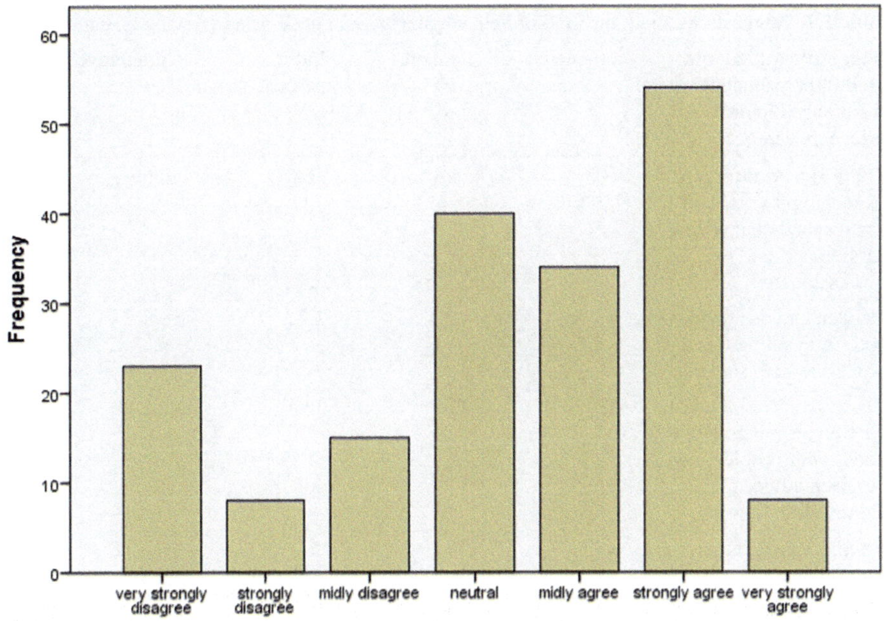

Fig. 5.7 I have friends with whom I can share my joys and sorrows

Table 5.6 Do you know where you would go to seek help on campus when grieving?

Do you know where you would go to seek help on campus when grieving?	Gender				Total	
	Males		Females			
	Freq	%	Freq	%	Freq	Total (%)
Yes	13	7	19	10	32	18
No	51	28	99	54	150	82
Total	64	36	118	64	182	100

5.4.3 *Ways to Improve the Quality of Life for Grieving Students*

Table 5.8 shows that the majority of students 39.6% (n-72) suggested that the university should establish more facilities to help those who are in need and 19.2% (n-35) indicated that the university should employ more professionals like counsellors, psychologists, and social workers to strengthen the support base. Ten point five percent (n-19) suggested that grieving students should just be given more emotional support, care and comfort and 7.1% (N-13) suggested that there should be programs established for grieving students to teach them how to overcome their challenges. Then 6.6% (N-12) suggested that there should be counselling sessions

Table 5.7 Suggestions about the kind of help students would need when grieving on campus

Suggestions about the kind of help students would need in order to grieve on campus	Frequency	Percent	Valid percent	Cumulative percent
There is a need for free psychologists, support groups, and counselling sessions offered by professionals	103	56.6	56.6	56.6
Reopen campus Guidance and Counselling Centre (GCU) to help students	4	2.2	2.2	58.8
There should be a place where you can go and talk about your problem and be given advice (i.e., Counselling Centre)	59	32.4	32.4	91.2
Enough books in our libraries	1	.5	.5	91.7
No suggestions	15	8.3	8.3	100.0
Total	182	100.0	100.0	

for the bereaved to help them cope with the situation and 6% (N-11) said the university should give financial assistance and bursaries as many students are from poor families. A 4.4% (N-8) suggested the university should open a social welfare department on campus or provide social caregivers to give assistance to the bereaved while another 4.4% (N-8) did not have any suggestions and 2.2% (N-4) suggested the university strengthens safety and security.

5.5 Discussion

The demographic data of the study consisted of one hundred and eight-two (182) respondents both males and females who were at undergraduate level and they were first year university students. Of the one hundred and eighty-two (182) respondents, there were one hundred and eighteen females (118) while there were sixty-four (64) males. All of them were Black Africans with the mean age of 25.5. The majority were single with a few cohabiting and one divorced. Most were living in the campus residence and a few were living outside the campus.

Table 5.8 Measures to be taken to improve the quality of life of grieving students on campus

Measures to be taken to improve the quality of life of grieving students on campus…	Frequency	Percent	Valid percent	Cumulative percent
Should establish more places of help for instance a counselling centre	72	39.6	39.6	39.6
Should employ more professionals like counsellors, psychologists, and social workers to increase support base	35	19.2	19.2	58.8
Strengthening safety and security should be prioritized	4	2.2	2.2	61.0
There should be programs established for grieving students to teach them how to overcome their challenges	13	7.1	7.1	68.1
Should give financial assistance and bursaries as many students are from poor families	11	6.0	6.0	74.1
There should be counselling sessions for the bereaved to help them cope with the situation	12	6.6	6.6	80.7
Just give them more emotional support, care and comfort	19	10.5	10.5	91.2
Should open social welfare department on campus or social caregivers to give assistance to the bereaved	8	4.4	4.4	95.6
No response	8	4.4	4.4	100.0
Total	182	100.0	100.0	

5.5.1 *Prevalence of Bereavement Amongst Students*

In terms of students understanding of bereavement findings show that students had somewhat similar understanding of what bereavement was. Most students understood it as loss of someone close, others understood it as loss of someone close through death while others understood it as when one has lost someone close. This finding is in line with Kail and Cavanaugh (2007) who defined bereavement as a state or condition caused by loss of someone through death. Students showed similar understanding as most of them understood that the significant part of bereavement is that the loss is of someone either close or related. Others understood it as an unhappy and painful emotion due to loss suffered, while others perceived it as understanding grief and how it affects individuals. After the loss, usually the bereaved experience grief manifesting different emotions such as anger, guilt, sadness, and sorrow due to loss suffered. This confirms what Kail and Cavanaugh (2007) observed, that the consequence of loss, in most cases, is followed by grief which could be viewed as the sorrow, hurt, anger, guilt, confusion, and other feelings that arise after suffering a loss through death.

The majority of students had suffered one or more losses of someone close to them through death in the past 24 months. This finding supports Servaty-Seib (2009) who argues that 22–30% of college undergraduates are likely to have experienced death of a family member or a friend in the previous year, and 35–48% are likely to be in their 24 months of grieving. This confirms what Balk (2001) has observed that as many as 48% of college undergraduates are in their first 24 months of grieving the death of a family member or a friend.

5.5.2 *Social Support Systems Available as Perceived by Grieving Students*

The findings show that most students had social support when they were grieving. Most students were getting social support either from family, friends, and any person or community who was willing to help. This finding correlated with the SCM which recognizes the importance of social support networks to help the bereaved persons to deal with the loss of loved ones. Furthermore, the SCM predicted that the bereaved students had important social support network such as family, friends and significant others who played a significant role in providing social support to the bereaved.

This finding was also supported Bath (2007) who observed that social support from family, friends, and colleagues was an important factor in the bereaved person's ability to cope after the loss of a loved one. This available support received by students can be explained by the fact that Africans value and embrace Ubuntu, by, among other things, supporting one another in times of stressful situations. After a family member has been lost through death there are gatherings by all family members, extended families, and even community in general. Therefore, the students have a social support network who offers tangible and emotional support when they need it. Cobb (1976) alluded in supporting this finding that social support is about showing others that one is loved and cared for, esteemed and valued, and part of a network of communication and mutual obligation. Cobb further argued that such information can come from a spouse or lover, other relatives, family, friends, social and community contacts such as churches, schools or other clubs.

5.5.3 The Help-Seeking Behavioral Patterns of Grieving Students' in Relation to Gender

The majority of female students did not know of any place on campus where they would go to and seek help when they grieve as compared to their male counterparts who were in the minority. The explanation for the discrepancy may be that females were the majority of students enrolled in the first year compared to their male counterparts. For the year 2013, all four faculties had enrolled 7093 first year students with 5018 females and 2075 males (Statistics supplied by Bureau for Institutional Research and Planning in 2013). This supports earlier findings at WSU by Qotoyi (2009) who found that a relatively small number of students utilized the services of Students' Guidance and Counselling (GCU) services. The impression is that students were either not fully aware of the existing service and value of such services or the new student orientation programmes were not as effective as they should be. Similarly Balk (2001) also observed that many college students would not turn to college counselling centre for help, and furthermore do not associate grief with mental health problem.

The majority of students suggested various kinds of help that students would need in order to grieve when on campus, implying that students should not be charged for services rendered by professionals. Some suggested a place where grieving students could go and talk about their problems and be given advice (i.e., a counselling centre). While others suggested that the university should reopen a Guidance and Counselling Unit, and the library. These findings are in line with Hardison, Niemeyer, and Lichstein (2005) who suggested that the efforts of the university should be directed toward familiarizing the student with the basic tasks of mourning and the emotional or psychological processes therein. This can be achieved by establishing places of help for the bereaved and enrolling properly trained professionals to help the bereaved students. Furthermore, the university should direct its efforts towards acquainting the students with the role of self-help groups (e.g. Compassionate Friends, Grief Support Group) among the bereaved as well as developing the students' appreciation of how various members of a health care team participate in the psychosocial need of patients and families at the time of death in an acute care setting (Hardison et al., 2005).

5.5.4 *Ways to Improve the Quality of Life for Grieving Students*

Students had different opinions and suggestions regarding measures that must be taken in order to improve the quality of life of grieving students on campus. The majority suggested that the university should establish more places for help suggesting counselling centres as an example. This finding correlated with Balk (2001) who argued that a university-based bereavement centre should be formed in order to coordinate and conduct coherent inquiry that fulfils the scholarly functions of discovery, application, and instruction. Some suggested that the university employ more professionals like counsellors, psychologists, and social workers to increase the support base, grieving students be given more emotional support, care and comfort and programs established to teach students how to cope with grief. This finding relates well with Balk (2001) who recommended training of non-bereaved students to provide peer support, to provide structured interventions for college students at risk of bereavement complications, to raise consciousness about bereavement on the university campus, and lastly, to conduct research into various bereavement populations and bereavement topics.

In addition to the above, other suggestions included; the university giving financial assistance and bursaries to students, a social welfare department being opened on campus, strengthening of safety and security. Qotoyi (2009) in his study also observed that WSU campuses were not safe, there was a lack of competent security resources which were of great concern. For instance, some academic staff members and students have either been robbed while in their offices or residences, others stabbed to death while being robbed, burglaries, students being raped, and motor vehicles being stolen. This lack of safety on campus can also have a negative impact on grieving students as they are always anxious and fearful.

5.6 Conclusions

The study serves as a platform to explore the plight suffered by first year students as they are the most vulnerable group of a university population. They are the ones who are confronted with plenty of challenges and difficulties. Most of the students come from different backgrounds, some come from rural backgrounds and it is their first time to be alone in another environment without their family. This becomes a problem because some of these students are introverts which make it difficult to make new friends at the university. So if these challenges cannot be dealt with as matter of urgency they can lead to disastrous situations such as academic dysfunction, high failure rate, non-attendance of classes, apathy in academic functions and dropouts, severe forms of grief or complicated grief, acute forms of depression and later major depression and even suicides. Therefore it is imperative that the university establishes policies aimed at improving and enhancing university community life after bereavement such as Bereavement Awareness Week. This also includes the establishment of Campus Support Groups to help the grieving students. In that way this will help to deter the negative impact of such loss on physiological, psychological and emotional wellbeing of grieving student, thus improving the quality of life of this population.

References

AIDS Foundation of South Africa. (2005). *HIV/AIDS prevalence: Trends and challenges*, p. 1 [Website selected briefs on line]. Retrieved July 25, 2006 from the World Wide Web: http://www.aids.org.za/hiv.htm.

Antonucci, T. C., Birditt, K. S., & Akiyama, H. (2009). Convoys of social relations: An interdisciplinary approach. In V. L. Bengston, D. Gans, N. M. Pulney, & M. Silverstein (Eds.), *Handbook of theories of aging* (2nd ed., pp. 247–260). New York: Springer.

Antonucci, T. C. (2001). Social relations: An examination of social networks, social support, and sense of control. In J. E. Birren & K. W. Schaie (Eds.), *Handbook of the psychology of aging* (5th ed., pp. 427–453). San Diego, CA: Academic Press.

Antonucci, T. C., & Akiyama, H. (1987). Social networks in adult life: A preliminary examination of the convoy model. *Journal of Gerontology, 42,* 519–527.

Balk, E. D. (2001). College student bereavement, scholarship, and the university: A call for university engagement. *Death Studies, 25*(1), 67–84.

Bath, D. M. (2007). No right words: Perceptions of grief and interactions with the bereaved. Manuscripts submitted for publication.

Bless, C., Smith, H., & Kagee, A. (2006). *Fundamentals of social research methods: An African perspective*. Cape Town: Juta.

Bowlby, J. (1969). *Attachment and loss*. New York: Basic Books.

Bowlby, J. (1982). Caring for children: Some influences on its development. In R. S. Cohen, S. H. Weissman, & B. J. Cohler (Eds.), *Parenthood*. New York: The Guilford Press.

Brannon, L. & Feist, J. (2004). *Health psychology: An introduction to behaviour and health* (5th ed.). Sydney: Wadsworth.

Bureau for Institutional Research and Planning. (2013). WSU *statistics for first year students in the year 2013*. Retrieved May 21, 2013, from http://www.wsu.ac.za/intranet/html.

Center for Disease Control and Prevention. (2006). *The Global HIV/AIDS Pandemic 2006*. Retrieved May 24, 2007, from http://www.cdc.gov/mmwr/preview/mmwrhtml/mm5531a1.html.

Cobb, S. (1976). Social support as a moderator of life stress. *Psychosomatic Medicine, 38,* 300–314.

Department of Health, South Africa. (2006). National HIV syphilis antenatal sero-prevalence survey in South Africa 2005. *Extrapolation of HIV Prevalence to the General Population*, p. 16 [Website selected briefs on line]. Retrieved July 25, 2006, from the World Wide Web http://www.doh.gov.za.

Fajgenbaum, D. (2007). College student bereavement: University responses, programs and policies, and recommendations for improvement. A published research thesis conducted in fulfillment of Honours in Human Science, Georgetown University.

Hardison, G. H., Neimeyer, A. R., & Lichstein, L. K. (2005). Insomnia and complicated grief symptoms in bereaved college students. *Journal of Behavioural Sleep Medicine, 3*(2), 99–111.

Hough, S. E., Magnan, A. M., Templin, T., & Gadelrab, F. H. (2005, July/August). Social network structure and social support in HIV-positive inner city mothers. *Journal of the Association of Nurses in AIDS Care, 16*(4), 14–24.

Kail, V. R., & Cavanaugh, C. J. (2007). *Human development: A life-span view* (4th ed.). London: Wadsworth.

Kahn, R. L., & Antonucci, T. C. (1980). Convoys over the life course: Attachment, roles and social support. In P. B. Baltes & O. G. Brim (Eds.), *Life-span development and behaviour* (pp. 253–286). New York: Academic Press.

Mead, G. H. (1934). *Mind, self, and society*. Chicago: Chicago University Press.

Merton, R. K. (1957). *Social theory and social structure*. Chicago: Free Press of Glencoe.

Moen, P. (2001). The gendered life course. In R. H. Binstock & L. K. George (Eds.), *Handbook of aging and the social sciences* (pp. 179–196). San Diego, CA, US: Academic Press.

Owens, S. (2003). African American women living with HIV/AIDS: Families as sources of support and of stress. *Social Work, 48,* 163–173.

Plath, D. W. (1980). *Long engagements: Maturity in modern Japan*. Stanford, CA: Stanford University Press.

Qotoyi, A. (2009). *Prevalence of academic stress among the Walter Sisulu University staff and students*. A dissertation submitted for partial fulfilment of Masters Degree in Industrial Psychology.

Servaty-Seib, H. L. (2009). Death of a friend during adolescence. In D. E. Balk & C. A. Corr (Eds.), *Adolescent encounters with death, bereavement, and coping* (pp. 217–235). New York: Springer.

Servaty-Seib, H. L., & Taub, D. J. (Eds.). (2008). *Assisting bereaved college students: New Directions for Students Services, Number 121*. New York: Jossey-Bass.

Sikkema, K. J., Hansen, N. B., Meade, C. S., Kochman, A., & Lee, R. S. (2005). Improvements in health-related quality of life following a group intervention for coping with AIDS bereavement among HIV infected men and women. *Quality of Life Research: An International Journal of Quality of Life Aspects of Treatment, Care and Rehabilitation, 14*(4), 991–1005.

Somhlaba, N. Z. (2006). Stress and coping in recent conjugally bereaved rural black spouses. Unpublished Doctoral Dissertation, University of Stellenbosch, South Africa.

Spangenberg, J. J., & Somhlaba, N. Z. (2003). *Stress and coping strategies in recent widowed rural black South African women*. Paper presented at the 8th European Congress of Psychology, Vienna, Austria, July 2003.

World Bank. (2005). *The World Bank Annual Report 2005: Year in Review*, Vol. 1. Washington, DC. © World Bank. https://openknowledge.worldbank.org/handle/10986/7537. License: CC BY 3.0 IGO.

World Health Organization. (2006). *Suicide prevention (SUPRE)*. Retrieved July 12, 2006, from http://www.who.int/mental_health/prevention/suicide/suicideprevention/print.html.

UNAIDS. (2006). *Report on the global HIV/AIDS epidemic: A UNAIDS 10th-anniversary special edition*. Geneva: Joint United Nations Programme on HIV/AIDS.

Zimet, G. D., Dahlem, N. W., Zimet, S. G., & Farley, G. K. (1988). The multidimensional scale of perceived social support (MSPSS). *Journal of Personality Assessment, 52,* 30–41.

Sabi Baninzi is a member of the faculty of Humanities, Social Science and Law in the Department of Psychology at Walter Sisulu University. He completed a Bachelor of Psychology Degree at Walter Sisulu University in 2010, then graduated in 2014 in Master of Arts in Psychology. He is also registered with Health Professions Council of South Africa (HPCSA) under the Board of Psychology as a Registered Psychological Counsellor including Board of Healthcare Funders (BHF). He has worked in different settings, including governmental departments (Department of Roads & Public Works working as Wellness Coordinator, Department of Justice & Constitutional Development as Family Counsellor, and Department of Health as Employee Assistance Programme (EAP) Practitioner); Non-Governmental Organizations (NGO's) which include the following Wellness Intervention Centre and Harambee working as Registered Psychological Counsellor. Currently, he is a Lecturer and Programme Coordinator for Student Registered Counsellor Programme at WSU. His work has been presented at the following conferences: International Society for Quality of Life Society (ISQOLS 2015), Population Association of Southern Africa (PASA 2015 & 2016), University of Venda & Walter Sisulu University-1st and 2nd UNIVEN International Research Conference 2015 & 2016, and Southern African Society for Education (SASE 2016). Currently, he is a registered Student Psychologist with HPCSA pursuing Masters in Clinical Psychology with Rhodes University.

Tembeka Mdleleni-Bookholane is a Senior Lecturer in the Department of Psychology, Faculty of Humanities, Social Sciences and Law at Walter Sisulu University (Nelson Mandela Drive-Campus) in the Eastern Cape Province in South Africa. She teaches Developmental Psychology, Community Psychology and Research Methodology. She has published the book: Death Through the Eyes of a Child.

Chapter 6
Community Well-Being Data Collection Methodology, the Case of Enschede, the Netherlands

Javier Martinez and Frans van den Bosch

Abstract The aim of this chapter is to describe the methodology of the data collection for the community well-being survey carried out in Enschede on behalf of the Community Well-being Institute, Seoul National University. We adapted "The Community Well-being Survey" questionnaire designed by the Community Well-being Institute for the study of six districts in Seoul, South Korea (Lee & Kim in Social factors and community well-being. Springer, pp. 13–37, 2016) to match it with the local context: the city of Enschede, the Netherlands. The methodology is explained as an example of how to collect well-being data.

Keywords Community well-being · Survey methods · Subjective well-being · Intersubjective well-being

6.1 Introduction

Enschede is located in the eastern part of the Netherlands close to the German border and is a medium sized city with 158,201 inhabitants by May 2015 (CBS, 2017). Enschede is subdivided into five administrative districts[1]: Noord, Oost, Zuid, West, and Centrum which encompass the main town and villages surrounding it including Boekelo, Glanerbrug and Lonneker (Fig. 6.1) and compromise a total of 68 neighbourhoods (Gemeente Enschede, 2017).

J. Martinez (✉) · F. van den Bosch
Faculty ITC—PGM, University of Twente, PO Box 217, 7500 AE Enschede, The Netherlands
e-mail: j.a.martinez@utwente.nl

F. van den Bosch
e-mail: fbosch@rsm.nl

[1] Enschede is also subdivided into ten statistical districts "*wijken*".

© Springer Nature Switzerland AG 2019

Y. Kee et al. (eds.), *Perspectives on Community Well-Being*, Community Quality-of-Life and Well-Being, https://doi.org/10.1007/978-3-030-15115-7_6

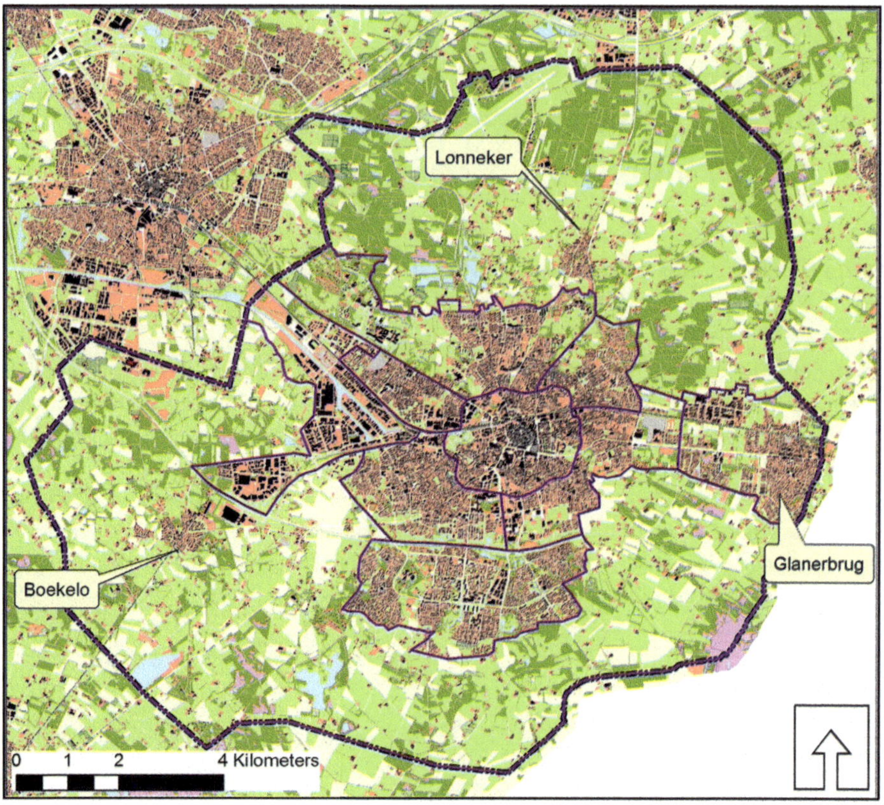

Fig. 6.1 Administrative boundary of the Municipality of Enschede (with villages)

Enschede had a booming textile industry until the 1970s. In the 1990s, several projects took place in different parts of Enschede in order to regenerate the city (Alarasi, Martinez, & Amer, 2016; Denters & Klok, 2010; van Melik, 2009). It is currently a service and knowledge intensive industry based city with the presence of many higher educational institutions.

This chapter first explains the adaptation of the questionnaire to suit the local context and the main characteristics and phases of the questionnaire administration. It is followed by a section describing the questionnaire administration and a section on the challenges presented in each part of the questionnaire. The last two sections deal with the data processing characteristics and conclusions including the potentials of analysing the questions spatially. The annex includes the English as well as the Dutch version of the questionnaire.

6.2 Questionnaire Adaptation to the Local Context

The original questionnaire was translated from English into Dutch.[2] The Dutch version was then adapted to the local context by checking the validity of the used categories (e.g. Dutch education levels) and cultural acceptability (e.g. questions related to religion, income). In order to facilitate comparability across different cities, the questionnaire was kept as much as possible in line with the one originally designed for the districts in Seoul city. A final version of the questionnaire was composed after several pilots, where iterations of the phrasing of questions, instructions to interviewers, and the order of questions had been fine-tuned and pre-tested.

The questionnaire is a compilation of four parts:

(1) Twenty-six questions about the level of satisfaction that the respondent has with (a) several aspects of his/her neighbourhood and (b) the same aspects when compared to the situation of other neighbourhoods[3];
(2) Ten questions related to the satisfaction to personal life;
(3) Eleven questions related to the community capitals and attachment; and
(4) Eleven questions on the socio-economic and demographic background of the respondent.

Based on the pilots, one of the most important change was introduced in the first part of the questionnaire. Since some of the facilities or aspects listed in the questionnaire were unknown to the participants we added the option "do not know, no opinion" as choice. Further details on these issues are explained later in this chapter within the section "Challenges and lessons learned from this first survey".

The questionnaire was also adapted in order to trace the geographical distribution of respondents and to facilitate spatial analysis. We included two questions to *geocode* the respondents. The interviewers asked the participants to provide the postcode of their home address. In the Netherlands, a four-digit postcode allows the identification of any neighbourhood and, with a six-digit code a unique street segment can be identified. The six-digit code in combination with the house number identifies the address. For obvious privacy and ethical reasons, we did not ask for a house number. Respondents were free to give a four or a six digit level postcode.

[2]The original Korean version of the questionnaire was translated into English by the Community Well-being Institute.

[3]According to Lee and Kim (2016) this element in the survey intends to capture **intersubjective community well-being** (CWB) which can be illustrated with the following example: "I may be dissatisfied with the level of traffic in my district, but at the same time I can be aware that the reason there is congestion in my district is because it is a desirable place to live. This is a relatively more objective way of thinking, because I can recognize the congestion as a given community parameter. At the same time, I can recognize that in comparison to other districts, my district is making adequate efforts for dealing with traffic congestion by placing police officers to direct traffic during rush hour. My satisfaction with the traffic situation can be different from my evaluation of it. We call the former (i.e. satisfaction) subjective CWB and the latter (i.e. evaluation) intersubjective CWB" (Lee & Kim, 2016, p. 20).

6.3 Questionnaire Administration

We used a mixed mode survey approach to conduct the survey (Bryman, 2016) and collected 106 responses. The questionnaire was administered through face-to-face structured interviews and online via the web (self-administered). Respondents could opt for either mode depending on their time availability. To reduce mode effects we used the same visual appearance in the survey design.

The respondents were selected using convenience sampling. Two interviewers visited a selection of public spaces located across Enschede (e.g. streets, squares, supermarket entrances, public library). They used tablets equipped with the questionnaire (SurveyMonkey® platform). A mix of public spaces had been identified to ascertain the addressing of potential respondents from the different social/economic groups (e.g., supermarkets at the low end range:—selling on average cheaper products—; mid-range and high-end range). The tablets had also a map with those public spaces loaded using Google maps. On average, each questionnaire took 30 min to complete and 30 min to recruit a person willing to participate.

To ensure a geographical balanced distribution of the participants we monitored the respondents per district. It should be noted that during the pilot phase it became clear that it would be very difficult to collect enough surveys in suburban areas of Enschede (e.g. the villages Boekelo or Lonneker, both at the outskirts of the Enschede municipality area—See Fig. 6.1). The main problem was to find local gathering areas where enough people would pass by. A door-to-door survey was discouraged since it is not a common practice in the Netherlands. The interviewers had to return to the field locations several times to find enough potential participants. In the city-centre, despite the large concentration of potential participants at gathering places (e.g. squares) and on the streets, the problem was to find people actually living in Enschede. Eventually the best locations to collect surveys where in front of (big) supermarkets, in front of the public city library and on the parking lots of local shopping centres.

6.3.1 Informed Consent and Strategy to Improve Response Rate

During the first two weeks, the interviewers tried to address passers-by on the street but many indicated that they did not want to participate in the survey, because of lack of time and the length of it.

To increase the response rate the approach towards potential respondents was enriched by using in the introduction of the questionnaire the "but you are free to accept or to refuse" technique (Gueguen & Pascual, 2005).

https://nl.surveymonkey.com/r/welzijn2015
WELZIJN
2015
UNIVERSITY OF TWENTE
Help ons met de verbetering van onze kennis over het welzijn in uw wijk.
We zijn benieuwd naar uw input, alvast bedankt voor het invullen van de enquête!
https://nl.surveymonkey.com/r/welzijn2015

Fig. 6.2 QR code card for participants willing to fill the survey at home, front/back side

Informed (oral) consent from all the participants was obtained using the following formulation:

> *"Sorry Madam/Sir, I have something to ask you* ***but you are free to accept or to refuse****. We are currently conducting a survey for the University of Twente on the perception of community well-being in Enschede. Would you accept to respond to a questionnaire that will take you 15–20 min?"*
>
> *[Note to interviewer: If the person refuses, thanks him/her. If he/she complies, the questionnaire will be administered].*

Due to time restrictions, some participants opted to complete the survey online from home. In those cases, the interviewers provided the participants with a business card shaped invitation containing the web address and a QR code linked to an online copy of the questionnaire, to complete the survey (Fig. 6.2).

6.4 Challenges in the Administration of the Questionnaire

The questionnaire is a compilation of four parts with a combination of closed-ended and open-ended questions and with different challenges that are discussed in the subsequent sections.

6.4.1 Part 1: Subjective Well-Being Versus Intersubjective Well-Being

The survey starts with twenty-six questions concerning the level of satisfaction that the respondent has with several aspects of his/her neighbourhood (aspects of community life such as public libraries, roads, etc.). Here the questions are grouped into two main categories. The first category relates to the **personal satisfaction levels** that pertain to community life on a 10-point Likert scale (subjective Community Well-being). For the second category, respondents have to **evaluate** the level of various aspects of community life on a 10-point Likert scale (intersubjective Community Well-being) by comparing the situation against other neighbourhoods.

In the case of Enschede, we found that some participants had difficulties to understand the following questions[4]:

Question 7b: many participants had no knowledge about the internet facilities in other neighbourhoods.

Questions 10, 11 and 13–15: if there was no public library or facilities for adult education in their neighbourhood participants answered: 'Do not know/no opinion'.

Question 16: in general, participants did not know the meaning of "general social services". The interviewers tried to name some examples like citizen service centre to explain what general social services are.

Question 19: many participants stated that you "could not know how well you are prepared for a disaster until it happens".

Questions 22–24: many participants were not aware about those aspects.

A quite substantial number of the respondents were not familiar with certain aspects in other parts of the city (e.g. waste collection service) when asked for evaluation them because, so as they said, "they do not come in other parts of the city". An indication of the total amount of respondents who did not know about other parts of the city can be inferred from Table 6.1. The column "difference follow up question" accounts for the difference between the total amount of respondents who answered "do not know" in the evaluation question (part b/intersubjective CWB) and those who answered "do not know" in the personal satisfaction level (part a/subjective CWB).

6.4.2 *Part 2: Individual Well-Being and Personal Life*

This part contains 10-point Likert scale questions related to individual well-being (IWB)[5] such as overall life satisfaction or to specific domains (e.g. health).

Some respondents found questions related to aspects of "your personal life" too personal and did not want to answer those due to privacy issues.

[4]Full questionnaire in English appears in Annex 1.

[5]For a discussion on the differences between subjective individual well-being (IWB), subjective and intersubjective community well-being (CWB) see Lee and Kim (2016).

Table 6.1 Difference follow up questions

Aspect	Difference follow up question
1. Overall living environment	7
2. Medical service	9
3. Waste collection service	19
4. Air quality	13
5. Green space	4
6. Public transportation	14
7. Internet service	11
8. Road quality	6
9. Culture and arts activities	9
10. Public library	2
11. Child friendly environment	9
12. Services for the elderly	10
13. Services for the disabled	7
14. Childcare services	13
15. General social services	5
16. Local public employee service and work ethic	8
17. Overall public services	8
18. Natural disaster preparedness	4
19. Public safety	9
20. Job training services	1
21. Management of city budget	5
22. Overall local economic conditions	5
23. Cost of living in your city	9

6.4.3 *Part 3: Community Capitals and Attachment*

This part contains one ranking question on the importance of different "capitals", and combination of 10-point Likert scale and open-ended questions mostly related to the level of attachment that the respondent had with the community. The main challenges of this part were related to *question 5* about "attachment". Participants often filled in 'Do not know/no opinion' because they do not participate in community activities or voluntary work. Some participants had problems ranking elements for the community well-being in their neighbourhood.

We found that some participants had difficulties to understand the following questions in particular:

Question 1: here the participants had to order the different elements (e.g. cultural capital, social capital). This was very difficult for them. It took a lot of time to first understand the question and second to establish a ranking.

Question 2, 3: about how people would describe a happy life or good life was easier. The interviewers had to summarize the answers because many participants described it in more than three words. The same issue also occurred with question 3: "What do you think is a nice area to live in or a nice neighbourhood?"

Question 4, 5, 7: In general, participants had no problems with the ratings (weak vs. strong),

Question 6: but they had difficulties describing why they had chosen a certain level. This issue also occurred with the following questions.

Question 9: When do you feel the strongest conflict or tensions with other residents?

Question 10: When do you feel the strongest sense of community or desire to cooperate with other residents? And

Question 11: How can we increase the level of trust in your neighbourhood?

6.4.4 Part 4: Objective Individual Well-Being

The last part of survey included questions on indicators of objective Individual Well-being (IWB). They were closed-end questions on demographic variables (sex, age, etc.) and other socio-economic variables and personal background characteristics such as income and religion.

In general, respondents had no problems in answering the questions except for two questions. The first one is *question 10* about the monthly income. In general, people in the Netherlands do not want to talk about how much money they earn. To avoid this, interviewers used the "but you are free to accept or to refuse" technique, or alternatively the interviewers offered the tablet to the participant so that he/she could choose the answer herself. The second issue was related to the economic class in *question 11*. Initially, it was very difficult for the participants to answer directly to which class they think they belong to. After a while, and to increase the speed of responses, the interviewers tried another technique; they formulated the class question twice; first by asking if they would belong to the highest, middle or lowest class. To gather a more precise outcome the interviewers asked: "do you belong to the top, middle or bottom of your previously indicated class." With these two answered the interviewers could fill in the exact class. This technique went well.

6.4.4.1 Data Process

All the responses were exported into SPSS® 23. Labels have been added to the variable values and translated back into English to facilitate future interpretation and analysis.

All the answers to open questions were translated from Dutch into English. For international comparisons, this can be a challenge as the adaptation to the local cultural context is often required. One example to illustrate this is that one respondent used an expression while using the local dialect referring to the sense of community but that it does not have a direct translation into English. The participant made use of the word "*noaberschap*" which refers to an old traditional expectation to help neighbouring farmers in your community.[6]

6.4.5 Spatial Analysis

The SPSS dataset was imported into a Geographic Information System (GIS) to map the distribution of responses by making use of the four and six digit postcode given as home address. Figures 6.3 and 6.4 illustrate the potential of mapping the different responses. Figure 6.3 overlays in one map the subjective CWB with the intersubjective CWB and includes those with no opinion. Figure 6.4 makes explicit the divergence between the subjective (a) and intersubjective CWB (b) with one district (in orange) showing a clear worse off evaluation compared to the personal satisfaction.

6.5 Conclusions

In this chapter, we described the methodology of the data collection for the community well-being survey carried out in Enschede between May and October 2015.

One of the most important steps before the data collection was to adapt the original questionnaire from Seoul to the context of Enschede.

In terms of the questionnaire design and implementation we found that the main problem encountered by some participants was the disability to differentiate between scoring in the Likert scale their own neighbourhood situation (personal satisfaction or subjective CWB) and then again scoring their own neighbourhood in relation to the rest of the city (evaluation or intersubjective CWB). Some respondents did not see the relation in the follow-up question (evaluation) and scored again their personal satisfaction (subjective CWB). In those cases, the interviewer had to explain the question to the respondent. This is an issue that in further versions of the survey should be considered, and in particular for online web surveys. An alternative way for addressing the difficulties in evaluating the aspects in intersubjective CWB would

[6]*Noaberschap* refers to the joint *noabers* (neighbours) in a small social, predominantly agricultural community. Within noaberschap applies the *Noaber* duty. This implies an obligation, for the neighbours (in a broad sense) to assist in word and deed if necessary. Traditionally it was a very large and intensive form of neighbourly assistance, which was essential for the occupants of farms and communities that cannot rely on good public facilities. Adapted and translated from https://nl.wikipedia.org/wiki/Noaberschap.

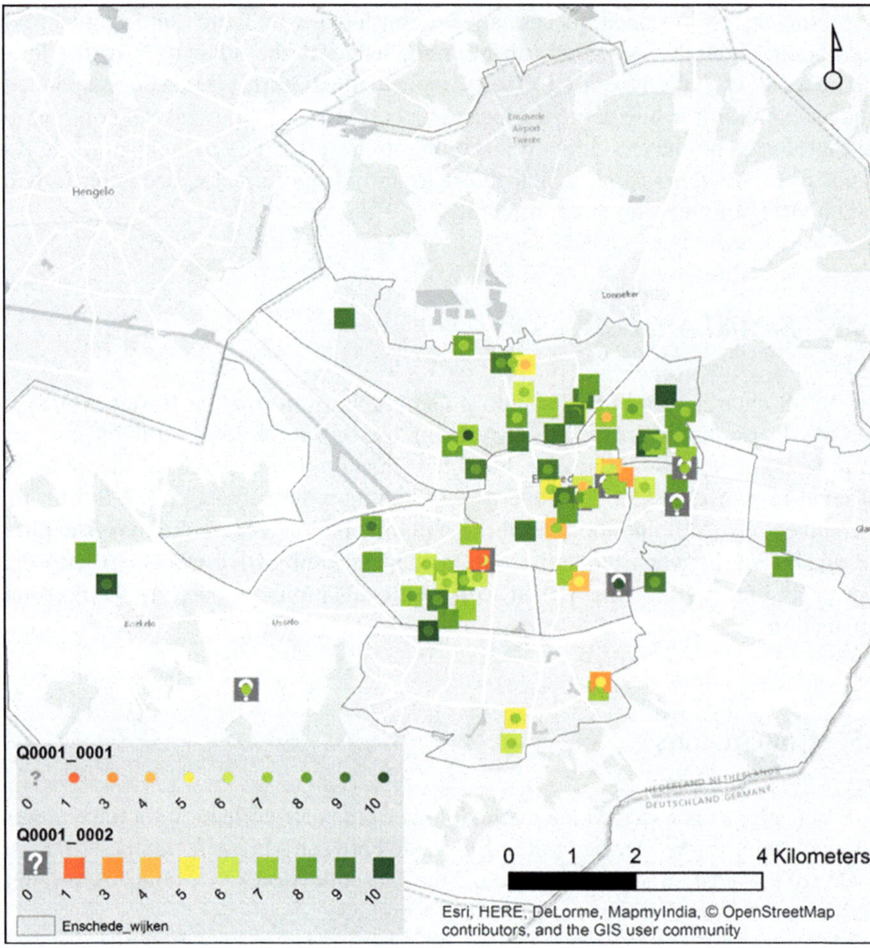

Fig. 6.3 Exploration of geographic variations of overall living environment satisfaction. Q0001_0001 refers to the personal satisfaction (subjective CWB) and Q0002_0002 refers to the evaluation (intersubjective CWB)

be to include a mid-point in the Likert scale defined as "no opinion". However, further research needs to be done to investigate the validity of such a measure for the concept of intersubjective well-being.

Finally, the inclusion of a question to geocode the respondents probed to be useful to present the spatial patterns of responses and to compare subjective and intersubjective responses.

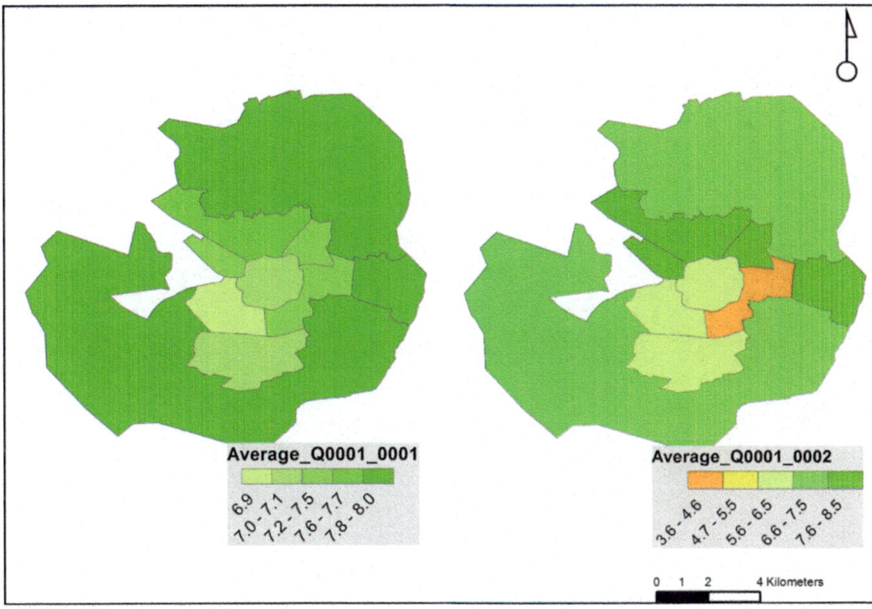

Fig. 6.4 Geographic variations of average overall living environment satisfaction at district level. **a** Personal satisfaction (subjective CWB) and **b** Evaluation (intersubjective CWB)

Acknowledgements This work was supported by the Ministry of Education of the Republic of Korea and the National Research Foundation of Korea (NRF-2016S1A3A2924563). We also would like to thank our two data collection assistants: Jan Engels and Floran Witting.

Annex 1—Original English Version Questionnaire

This questionnaire was developed and revised by Community Wellbeing Institute and Global Community Institute

[Part 1]

The following questions are about various aspects of *your city*. For each item, please indicate your *personal level of satisfaction* on the *left* hand side and *evaluation compared to other cities* on the *right* hand side, where "1" is the lowest level of satisfaction or evaluation and "10" is the highest level of satisfaction or evaluation.

Personal satisfaction											Evaluation									
Very high		Slightly high				Slightly low		Very low			Very low			Slightly low			Slightly high			Very high
10	9	8	7	6	5	4	3	2	1	1. Overall living environment	1	2	3	4	5	6	7	8	9	10
10	9	8	7	6	5	4	3	2	1	2. Medical service	1	2	3	4	5	6	7	8	9	10
10	9	8	7	6	5	4	3	2	1	3. Waste collection service	1	2	3	4	5	6	7	8	9	10
10	9	8	7	6	5	4	3	2	1	4. Air quality	1	2	3	4	5	6	7	8	9	10
10	9	8	7	6	5	4	3	2	1	5. Green space	1	2	3	4	5	6	7	8	9	10
10	9	8	7	6	5	4	3	2	1	6. Public transportation	1	2	3	4	5	6	7	8	9	10
10	9	8	7	6	5	4	3	2	1	7. Internet service	1	2	3	4	5	6	7	8	9	10
10	9	8	7	6	5	4	3	2	1	8. Road quality	1	2	3	4	5	6	7	8	9	10
10	9	8	7	6	5	4	3	2	1	9. Culture and arts activities	1	2	3	4	5	6	7	8	9	10
10	9	8	7	6	5	4	3	2	1	10. Public library	1	2	3	4	5	6	7	8	9	10
10	9	8	7	6	5	4	3	2	1	11. Lifelong education service	1	2	3	4	5	6	7	8	9	10
10	9	8	7	6	5	4	3	2	1	12. Educational environment	1	2	3	4	5	6	7	8	9	10
10	9	8	7	6	5	4	3	2	1	13. Services for the elderly	1	2	3	4	5	6	7	8	9	10
10	9	8	7	6	5	4	3	2	1	14. Services for the disabled	1	2	3	4	5	6	7	8	9	10

(continued)

(continued)

Personal satisfaction											Evaluation									
Very high		Slightly high				Slightly low		Very low			Very low			Slightly low			Slightly high			Very high
10	9	8	7	6	5	4	3	2	1	15. Childcare services	1	2	3	4	5	6	7	8	9	10
10	9	8	7	6	5	4	3	2	1	16. General social services	1	2	3	4	5	6	7	8	9	10
10	9	8	7	6	5	4	3	2	1	17. Local public employee service and work ethic	1	2	3	4	5	6	7	8	9	10
10	9	8	7	6	5	4	3	2	1	18. Overall public services	1	2	3	4	5	6	7	8	9	10
10	9	8	7	6	5	4	3	2	1	19. Natural disaster preparedness	1	2	3	4	5	6	7	8	9	10
10	9	8	7	6	5	4	3	2	1	20. Public safety	1	2	3	4	5	6	7	8	9	10
10	9	8	7	6	5	4	3	2	1	21. Police force	1	2	3	4	5	6	7	8	9	10
10	9	8	7	6	5	4	3	2	1	22. Job training services	1	2	3	4	5	6	7	8	9	10
10	9	8	7	6	5	4	3	2	1	23. Support for the unemployed	1	2	3	4	5	6	7	8	9	10
10	9	8	7	6	5	4	3	2	1	24. Management of city budget	1	2	3	4	5	6	7	8	9	10
10	9	8	7	6	5	4	3	2	1	25. Overall local economic conditions	1	2	3	4	5	6	7	8	9	10
10	9	8	7	6	5	4	3	2	1	26. Cost of living in your city	1	2	3	4	5	6	7	8	9	10

[Part 2]

The following questions are about various aspects of *your personal life*. Please indicate the level of each item where "1" is the lowest level and "10" is the highest level.

	Very low			Slightly low			Slightly high			Very high
1. Overall **life satisfaction**	1	2	3	4	5	6	7	8	9	10
2. Satisfaction with **your health**	1	2	3	4	5	6	7	8	9	10
3. Satisfaction with **your job/occupation**	1	2	3	4	5	6	7	8	9	10
4. Satisfaction with **your cultural activity**	1	2	3	4	5	6	7	8	9	10
5. Satisfaction with your participation in **local community activity**	1	2	3	4	5	6	7	8	9	10
6. Satisfaction with your level of participation in **volunteer activity**	1	2	3	4	5	6	7	8	9	10
7. Satisfaction with the **amount of local taxes** you pay	1	2	3	4	5	6	7	8	9	10
8. **Trust** in **others**	1	2	3	4	5	6	7	8	9	10
9. **Trust in local government**	1	2	3	4	5	6	7	8	9	10
10. **Trust** in **national government**	1	2	3	4	5	6	7	8	9	10

[Part 3]

For the following items, please write down your answers in your own words or circle your answer.

1. How important are the following elements for community well-being? Please rank the items in order of importance where "**1**" is the **least important** and "**6**" is the **most important**.
   ( ) Cultural Capital, such as leisure, art, heritage, ethnicity, and shared knowledge.
   ( ) Social Capital, such as trust, commitment, community bonding, mutual help.
   ( ) Human Capital, such as labor, education, and health.
   ( ) Economic Capital, such as financial assets.
   ( ) Physical Capital, such as natural environment, built environment.
   ( ) Political Capital, such as equity, representation, access, political participation.
2. How would you describe a **happy life** or **good life**? Please give us 3 descriptions.
   (1)________________________ (2)________________________
   (3)______________________________.
3. What do you think is a **nice area to live in** or **a nice neighborhood**? Please give us 3 descriptions.
   (1)______________________________
   (2)______________________________
   (3)______________________________.
4. How strong or weak are your desires to continue to live in this city?

WEAK		<---------		Desire to live here			-------->		STRONG
□①	□②	□③	□④	□⑤	□⑥	□⑦	□⑧	⑨	□⑩

5. How strong or weak is your sense of attachment to this city? Sense of attachment means identifying with the city as "my neighborhood" or identifying yourself as a ("INCLUDE APPROPRIATE TERM, e.g. New Yorker, San Franciscan, etc.").

WEAK		<---------		Sense of Attachment			-------->		STRONG
□①	□②	□③	□④	□⑤	□⑥	□⑦	□⑧	⑨	□⑩

6. In the previous question, what motivated you to choose that level of attachment?
   ____.
7. How strong or weak is your intention to participate in local community activities?

WEAK		<---------		Intention to participate			-------->		STRONG
□①	□②	□③	□④	□⑤	□⑥	□⑦	□⑧	⑨	□⑩

8. In the previous question, what motivated your intention to participate?
   ____.
9. When do you feel **the strongest conflict** or **tensions** with other residents of your city?
   ____.
10. When do you feel **the strongest sense of community** or **desire to cooperate** with other residents of your city?
    ____.

11. How can we increase the level of trust in our city?

____.

[Part 4]

The following questions ask about your personal background. This information will be used only for research and we ask for your accurate responses.

1. Gender (1) Male [] (2) Female [].
2. Age [__] years old.
3. Religious background (1) Protestant [] (2) Catholic [] (3) Buddhist [] (4) Muslim [] (5) Not religious [] (6) Other [Please explain: ______________________].
4. How long have you lived in this city? (Regardless of formal documents) [] years.
5. Which of the following best describes your living quarter? (1) I own the house [] (2) I rent the house [] (3) I live in a multiunit house [] (4) Other [Please explain: ______________________].
6. Which of the following best describes your current marital status? (1) Single-never married [] (2) Married [] (Includes common law marriage, weekend/long distance marriage, and nursing home) (3) Separated or divorced [].
7. Excluding yourself, how many family members (including adults and children) do you currently live with? [__] persons.
8. What is your highest level of education? (1) Less than elementary school graduate [] (2) Middle school graduate [] (3) High school graduate [] (4) University or community college graduate [] (5) Graduate school or higher [].
9. Which of the following best describes your current occupation status? (1) Wage employee [] (2) Self-employed without other employees [] (3) Self-employed with other employees [] (4) Employee of family business without pay [] (5) Currently searching for a job, but not employed [].
10. On average, what was your monthly household income in the past year (in USD)? (1) Less than 3000 [] (2) 3001–4999 [] (3) 5000–6999 [] (4) 7000–8999 [] (5) 9000–10,999 [] (6) 11,000–12,999 [] (7) 13,000–14,999 [] (8) 15,000–16,999 [] (9) 17,000–18,999 [] (10) 19,000–20,999 [] (11) 21,000–22,999 [] (12) 23,000–24,999 [] (13) Monthly average USD 25,000 or more [].
11. Which socioeconomic class do you think you are a part of? Please circle the corresponding number. For example, circle "1" for the lowest group and "9" for the highest group.

Low			Middle			High		
Low	Middle	High	Low	Middle	High	Low	Middle	High
(1) []	(2) []	(3) []	(4) []	(5) []	(6) []	(7) []	(8) []	(9) []

Annex 2—Dutch Version Questionnaire. Opening Page and Subsequent Pages (Screenshots from SurveyMonkey®)

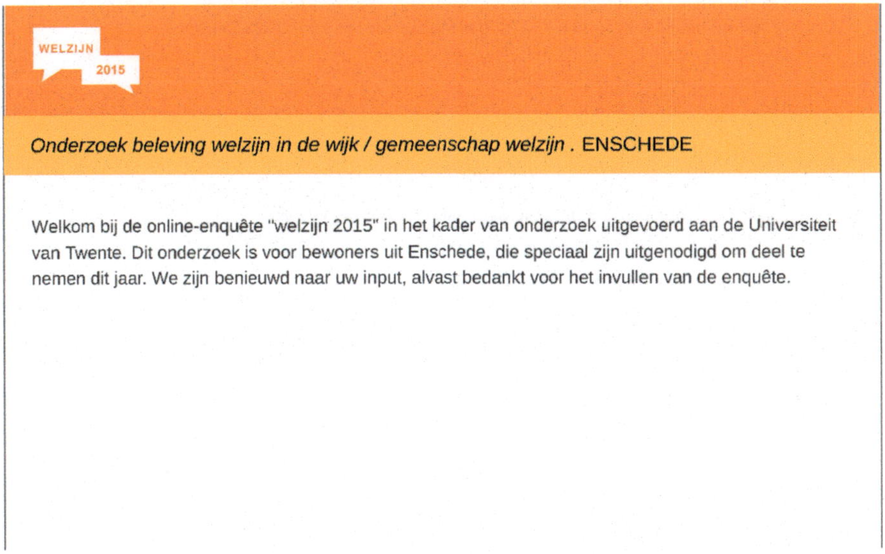

WELZIJN 2015

Onderzoek beleving welzijn in de wijk / gemeenschap welzijn . ENSCHEDE

Welkom bij de online-enquête "welzijn 2015" in het kader van onderzoek uitgevoerd aan de Universiteit van Twente. Dit onderzoek is voor bewoners uit Enschede, die speciaal zijn uitgenodigd om deel te nemen dit jaar. We zijn benieuwd naar uw input, alvast bedankt voor het invullen van de enquête.

WELZIJN 2015

Onderzoek beleving welzijn in de wijk / gemeenschap welzijn . ENSCHEDE

De volgende vragen gaan over verschillende aspecten van uw wijk.

Voor elk item kunt U aangeven wat uw persoonlijke mate van tevredenheid is.

a- Eerst geeft U uw persoonlijke waardering van aspecten van uw eigen wijk.
b- Daarna scoort U dezelfde aspect, waarbij U uw eigen wijk vergelijkt met de rest van uw stad.

Het laagste niveau van tevredenheid is "1" en het hoogste is "10".

	1(Heel laag)	2	3	4(Redelijk laag)	5	6	7(Redelijk hoog)	8	9	10(Heel hoog)	Weet niet/geen mening
1a.De totale leefomgeving (eigen wijk)	○	○	○	○	○	○	○	○	○	○	○
1b.De totale leefomgeving (in vergelijking met de rest van de stad)	○	○	○	○	○	○	○	○	○	○	○
2a.Medische voorzieningen	○	○	○	○	○	○	○	○	○	○	○
2b.Medische voorzieningen	○	○	○	○	○	○	○	○	○	○	○
3a. Afvalinzameling	○	○	○	○	○	○	○	○	○	○	○
3b. Afvalinzameling	○	○	○	○	○	○	○	○	○	○	○
4a.Luchtkwaliteit	○	○	○	○	○	○	○	○	○	○	○
4b.Luchtkwaliteit	○	○	○	○	○	○	○	○	○	○	○
5a.Groene ruimte	○	○	○	○	○	○	○	○	○	○	○
5b.Groene ruimte	○	○	○	○	○	○	○	○	○	○	○

2

WELZIJN 2015

Onderzoek beleving welzijn in de wijk / gemeenschap welzijn . ENSCHEDE

a- Eerst geeft U uw persoonlijke waardering van aspecten van uw eigen wijk.
b- Daarna scoort U dezelfde aspect, waarbij U uw eigen wijk vergelijkt met de rest van uw stad.
Het laagste niveau van tevredenheid is "1" en het hoogste is "10".

	1(Heel laag)	2	3	4(Redelijk laag)	5	6	7(Redelijk hoog)	8	9	10(Heel hoog)	Weet niet/geen mening
6a.Openbaar vervoer (eigen wijk)	○	○	○	○	○	○	○	○	○	○	○
6b.Openbaar vervoer (in vergelijking met de rest van de stad)	○	○	○	○	○	○	○	○	○	○	○
7a.Internet voorzieningen	○	○	○	○	○	○	○	○	○	○	○
7b.Internet voorzieningen	○	○	○	○	○	○	○	○	○	○	○
8a. Kwaliteit wegen en straten	○	○	○	○	○	○	○	○	○	○	○
8b. Kwaliteit wegen en straten	○	○	○	○	○	○	○	○	○	○	○
9a.Culturele activiteiten	○	○	○	○	○	○	○	○	○	○	○
9b.Culturele activiteiten	○	○	○	○	○	○	○	○	○	○	○
10a.Openbare bibliotheek	○	○	○	○	○	○	○	○	○	○	○
10b.Openbare bibliotheek	○	○	○	○	○	○	○	○	○	○	○

3

WELZIJN 2015

Onderzoek beleving welzijn in de wijk / gemeenschap welzijn . ENSCHEDE

a- Eerst geeft U uw persoonlijke waardering van aspecten van uw eigen wijk.
b- Daarna scoort U dezelfde aspect, waarbij U uw eigen wijk vergelijkt met de rest van uw stad.
Het laagste niveau van tevredenheid is "1" en het hoogste is "10".

	1(Heel laag)	2	3	4(Redelijk laag)	5	6	7(Redelijk hoog)	8	9	10(Heel hoog)	Weet niet/geen mening
11a. Voorzieningen voor onderwijs voor volwassenen en cursussen (bv. Volksuniversiteit) (eigen wijk)	○	○	○	○	○	○	○	○	○	○	○
11b. Voorzieningen voor onderwijs voor volwassenen en cursussen (bv. Volksuniversiteit) (in vergelijking met de rest van de stad)	○	○	○	○	○	○	○	○	○	○	○
12a. Kindvriendelijke omgeving	○	○	○	○	○	○	○	○	○	○	○
12b. Kindvriendelijke omgeving	○	○	○	○	○	○	○	○	○	○	○
13a. Voorzieningen voor ouderen	○	○	○	○	○	○	○	○	○	○	○
13b. Voorzieningen voor ouderen	○	○	○	○	○	○	○	○	○	○	○
14a. Voorzieningen voor gehandicapten	○	○	○	○	○	○	○	○	○	○	○
14b. Voorzieningen voor gehandicapten	○	○	○	○	○	○	○	○	○	○	○
15a. Voorzieningen kinderopvang	○	○	○	○	○	○	○	○	○	○	○
15b. Voorzieningen kinderopvang	○	○	○	○	○	○	○	○	○	○	○

4

WELZIJN 2015

Onderzoek beleving welzijn in de wijk / gemeenschap welzijn . ENSCHEDE

a- Eerst geeft U uw persoonlijke waardering van aspecten van uw eigen wijk.
b- Daarna scoort U dezelfde aspect, waarbij U uw eigen wijk vergelijkt met de rest van uw stad.

Het laagste niveau van tevredenheid is "1" en het hoogste is "10".

	1(Heel laag)	2	3	4(Redelijk laag)	5	6	7(Redelijk hoog)	8	9	10(Heel hoog)	Weet niet/geen mening
16a.Algemene sociale voorzieningen (eigen wijk)	○	○	○	○	○	○	○	○	○	○	○
16b.Algemene sociale voorzieningen (in vergelijking met de rest van de stad)	○	○	○	○	○	○	○	○	○	○	○
17a.Waardering voor medewerkers van lokale voorzieningen	○	○	○	○	○	○	○	○	○	○	○
17a. Waardering voor medewerkers van lokale voorzieningen	○	○	○	○	○	○	○	○	○	○	○
18b.Algemene openbare voorzieningen	○	○	○	○	○	○	○	○	○	○	○
18b.Algemene openbare voorzieningen	○	○	○	○	○	○	○	○	○	○	○
19a. Voorbereiding op (natuur) rampen	○	○	○	○	○	○	○	○	○	○	○
19b. Voorbereiding op (natuur) rampen	○	○	○	○	○	○	○	○	○	○	○
20a. Openbare veiligheid	○	○	○	○	○	○	○	○	○	○	○
20b. Openbare veiligheid	○	○	○	○	○	○	○	○	○	○	○

WELZIJN 2015

Onderzoek beleving welzijn in de wijk / gemeenschap welzijn . ENSCHEDE

a- Eerst geeft U uw persoonlijke waardering van aspecten van uw eigen wijk.
b- Daarna scoort U dezelfde aspect, waarbij U uw eigen wijk vergelijkt met de rest van uw stad.

Het laagste niveau van tevredenheid is "1" en het hoogste is "10".

	1(Heel laag)	2	3	4(Redelijk laag)	5	6	7(Redelijk hoog)	8	9	10(Heel hoog)	Weet niet/geen mening
21a.Politie (eigen wijk)	○	○	○	○	○	○	○	○	○	○	○
21b.Politie (in vergelijking met de rest van de stad)	○	○	○	○	○	○	○	○	○	○	○
22a. Voorzieningen voor Arbeidstraining	○	○	○	○	○	○	○	○	○	○	○
22b. Voorzieningen voor Arbeidstraining	○	○	○	○	○	○	○	○	○	○	○
23a. Ondersteuning werklozen (bv. UWV)	○	○	○	○	○	○	○	○	○	○	○
23b. Ondersteuning werklozen (bv. UWV)	○	○	○	○	○	○	○	○	○	○	○
24a. Beheer stedelijk begroting	○	○	○	○	○	○	○	○	○	○	○
24b. Beheer stedelijk begroting	○	○	○	○	○	○	○	○	○	○	○
25a.Algehele lokale economische omstandigheden	○	○	○	○	○	○	○	○	○	○	○
25b.Algehele lokale economische omstandigheden	○	○	○	○	○	○	○	○	○	○	○
26a. Kosten van levensonderhoud	○	○	○	○	○	○	○	○	○	○	○
26b. Kosten van levensonderhoud	○	○	○	○	○	○	○	○	○	○	○

6

WELZIJN 2015

Onderzoek beleving welzijn in de wijk / gemeenschap welzijn . ENSCHEDE

De volgende vragen gaan over verschillende aspecten van je persoonlijke leven. Wij vragen U het niveau van tevredenheid aan te geven. Het laagste niveau is 1 en '10' het hoogste.

	1(Heel laag)	2	3	4(redelijk laag)	5	6	7(redelijk hoog_	8	9	10(Heel hoog)	Weet niet/geen mening
1. De algehele tevredenheid met uw leven											
2. Tevredenheid met uw gezondheid											
3. Tevredenheid met uw baan / beroep											
4. Tevredenheid met uw culturele activiteiten											
5. Tevredenheid met uw deelname aan de lokale gemeenschapsactiviteiten											
6. Tevredenheid met uw mate van deelname aan vrijwilligerswerk											
7. Tevredenheid met de hoogte van de lokale belastingen die U betaalt											
8. Vertrouwen in anderen											
9. Vertrouwen in de lokale overheid											
10. Vertrouwen in de nationale regering											

7

WELZIJN 2015

Onderzoek beleving welzijn in de wijk / gemeenschap welzijn . ENSCHEDE

Hoe belangrijk zijn de volgende elementen voor het welzijn van de gemeenschap in uw wijk?
Rangschik de items in volgorde van belangrijkheid, waarbij "1" het minst belangrijk is en "6" de belangrijkste.

	1(minst belangrijk)	2	3	4	5	6(belangrijkste)
Cultureel elementen, zoals recreatie, kunst, erfgoed, etnische en kulturele diversiteit, en gedeelde kennis	○	○	○	○	○	○
Sociaal elementen, zoals vertrouwen, betrokkenheid, binding met gemeenschap, onderlinge hulpvaardigheid	○	○	○	○	○	○
Menselijk elementen, zoals arbeid, onderwijs en gezondheidszorg	○	○	○	○	○	○
Economisch elementen, zoals financieel bezit	○	○	○	○	○	○
Materieel elementen, zoals natuurlijke omgeving, gebouwen	○	○	○	○	○	○
Politiek elementen, zoals gelijkheid, vertegenwoordiging, toegankelijkheid, politieke participatie	○	○	○	○	○	○

Hoe zou U een gelukkig leven of goed leven omschrijven? Geef 3 woorden of korte beschrijvingen.

1-

2-

3-

8

Hoe zou U een mooi gebied om te wonen of een leuke buurt omschrijven? Geef 3 woorden of korte beschrijvingen.

1-

2-

3-

Hoe sterk of zwak is uw verlangen om in deze stad te (blijven) wonen?
1= Zwak
10= Sterk

	1(Zwak)	2	3	4	5	6	7	8	9	10(Sterk)
Verlangen om hier te wonen	○	○	○	○	○	○	○	○	○	○

Hoe sterk of zwak is uw gevoel van verbondenheid met deze wijk?

	1(Zwak)	2	3	4	5	6	7	8	9	10(Sterk)
Gevoel van verbondenheid	○	○	○	○	○	○	○	○	○	○

Beschrijf kort waarom U bij vorige vraag hebt gekozen voor een bepaald niveau van verbondenheid.

Hoe sterk of zwak is uw voornemen om deel te nemen aan de lokale gemeenschapsactiviteiten?

	1(Zwak)	2	3	4	5	6	7	8	9	10(Sterk)
Voornemen om deel te nemen	○	○	○	○	○	○	○	○	○	○

Beschrijf kort waarom U bij vorige vraag hebt gekozen voor een bepaald niveau van voornemen.

Wanneer heb je of ervaar je de grootste conflicten of spanningen met andere bewoners van je wijk?

Wanneer heb je het sterkste gevoel van gemeenschap of de wens om samen te werken met andere bewoners van je wijk?

Hoe kan uw vertrouwen in de wijk versterkt worden?

WELZIJN 2015

Onderzoek beleving welzijn in de wijk / gemeenschap welzijn . ENSCHEDE

De volgende vragen gaan over uw persoonlijke achtergrond. Deze informatie zal alleen gebruikt worden voor onderzoek en we verzoeken U de vragen nauwkeurig te beantwoorden.

Geslacht

- ◯ Man
- ◯ Vrouw

Wat is uw geboortejaar (bijvoorbeeld 1975)

[ ]

Levensbeschouwelijke achtergrond

- ◯ Protestants
- ◯ Rooms-Katholiek
- ◯ Boeddhistisch
- ◯ Moslim
- ◯ Joods
- ◯ Hindoe
- ◯ Geen
- ◯ Overige. Namelijk:

[ ]

Hoe lang woon je in deze wijk?

Jaar [ ]

Wat is op U van toepassing?:

- ◯ Ik woon in een huis
- ◯ Ik woon in een flat of appartement
- ◯ Ik woon op kamers (bijv. bij particulier of studentenhuisvesting)
- ◯ Overige. Toelichting:

[ ]

10

Wat is op U van toepassing?:

◯ Ik ben de eigenaar

◯ Ik ben huurder

Hoe is uw huishouden samen gesteld?

◯ Gehuwd of samenwonend zonder thuiswonende kinderen

◯ Gehuwd of samenwonend met thuiswonende kinderen

◯ Eénouder-huishouden

◯ Alleenstand

◯ Anders

Met hoeveel familieleden (waaronder volwassenen en kinderen) woont U momenteel?

Personen [ ]

Wat is uw hoogst genoten opleiding?

◯ Minder dan voortgezet gewoon lager onderwijs (basisonderwijs, lagere school

◯ Lager onderwijs (basisonderwijs, lagere school

◯ Lbo of vso (lts, leao, vbo, huishoudschool, ambachtsschool)

◯ Vmbo of lwoo (inclusief theoretische leerweg)

◯ Mavo (ulo, mulo)

◯ Havo (mms)

◯ Vwo, gymnasium of atheneum (hbs, lyceum)

◯ MBO (b.v. MTS, MEAO, UTS)

◯ HBO

◯ Wetenschappelijk onderwijs (Universiteit)

Welke van onderstaande arbeidsomstandigheden is/zijn op U van toepassing?

◯ In loondienst

◯ Zelfstandige zonder andere werknemers

◯ Zelfstandige met andere werknemers

◯ AOW/gepensioneerd

◯ Werk zoekend

11

Wat was (gemiddeld) het bruto maandinkomen van uw huishouden in het afgelopen jaar (in euro's)?

- ◯ (1) minder dan 1000
- ◯ (2) 1.001-1.999
- ◯ (3) 2.000- 2.499
- ◯ (4) 2.500 -2.999
- ◯ (5) 3.000 - 3.499
- ◯ (6) 3.500 - 3.999
- ◯ (7) 4.000 – of meer

Tot welke sociaal-economische klasse denkt U te behoren? waarbij "1" de laagste is en "9" de hoogste.

- ◯ 1 Laag
- ◯ 2 (Laag-Midden)
- ◯ 3 (Laag-Hoog)
- ◯ 4 (Midden-Laag)
- ◯ 5 Midden
- ◯ 6 (Midden-Hoog)
- ◯ 7 (Hoog-Laag)
- ◯ 8 (Hoog-Midden)
- ◯ 9 Hoog

Wat is uw postcode vier cijfer? (bijvoorbeeld: 1234)

[ ]

Wat zijn uw postcode twee letters? (bijvoorbeeld: AB)

[ ]

Dit is het einde van de vragenlijst. HARTELIJK DANK VOOR UW MEDEWERKING!
Hier kunt U uw eventuele opmerkingen kwijt over de vragenlijst

[ ]

12

References

Alarasi, H., Martinez, J., & Amer, S. (2016). Children's perception of their city centre. A qualitative GIS methodological investigation in a Dutch city. *Children's Geographies, 14*(4), 437–452. https://doi.org/10.1080/14733285.2015.1103836.

Bryman, A. (2016). *Social research methods* (5th ed.). Oxford and New York: Oxford University Press.

CBS. (2017). Bevolkingsontwikkeling; regio per maand. CBS. http://statline.cbs.nl.

Denters, B., & Klok, P. J. (2010). Rebuilding roombeek: Patterns of citizen participation in Urban governance. *Urban Affairs Review, 45*(5), 583–607. https://doi.org/10.1177/1078087409356756.

Gemeente Enschede. (2017). Stadsdelen, wijken en dorpen. Retrieved from https://www.enschede.nl/.

Gueguen, N., & Pascual, A. (2005). Improving the response rate to a street survey: An evaluation of the "but you are free to accept or to refuse" technique. *Psychological Record, 55*(2), 297–303.

Lee, S. J., & Kim, Y. (2016). Structure of well-being: An exploratory study of the distinction between individual well-being and community well-being and the importance of intersubjective community well-being. *Social Factors and Community Well-Being*, 13–37. Springer.

van Melik, R. (2009). Visualising the effect of private-sector involvement on redeveloped public spaces in the Netherlands. *Tijdschrift voor Economische en Sociale Geografie, 100*(1), 114–120. https://doi.org/10.1111/j.1467-9663.2009.00512.x.

Javier Martinez is Assistant Professor in the Department of Urban and Regional Planning and Geo-Information Management within the Faculty of Geo-Information Science and Earth Observation (ITC), University of Twente, the Netherlands. He is also coordinator of the Urban Planning and Management specialization of the 2-year Master's degree in Geo-Information Science and Earth Observation. He graduated as an architect from the Faculty of Architecture, Planning and Design of Rosario National University (UNR), Argentina, and obtained his MSc degree in Geo-Information for Urban Planning from ITC. He received his PhD from the Faculty of Geosciences, Utrecht University, for his thesis Monitoring intra-urban inequalities with GIS-based indicators: with a case study in Rosario, Argentina. Between 1999 and 2001, he worked in Argentina in the Office of Strategic Planning in Rosario (PER) designing its Urban Indicators System. His research, publications and training experience are focused on the application of GIS, mixed methods and indicators for policy-making, urban poverty, and quality-of-life and intra-urban inequalities. From 2010 up until November 2014 he was co-coordinator of the Network-Association of European Researchers on Urbanization in the South (N-AERUS). Since 2017, he has been a member of the board of directors of the International Society of Quality of Life Studies (ISQOLS).

Ing. Frans van den Bosch studied informatics and has over 25 years of experience in applying Geographic Information Science for Urban related applications. He executes a variety of tasks in the field of education, research and consultancy at the Department of Urban and Regional Planning and Geo-Information Management at ITC, University of Twente. His main research interests are in (transport) systems modelling and analysis with advanced GIS-based spatial analytical methods, modelling techniques and the development of collaborative spatial decision support systems in urban planning.

Chapter 7
The Relationship Between the Types of Needs Satisfaction and Subjective Well-Being

Young Woong Kang and Seung Jong Lee

Abstract The purpose of this study is to clarify the relationship between satisfaction type of residents' needs and subjective well-being. For this analysis, the organization conducts ranked logistic analysis using the 2017 Community Well-Being Survey of Korea. The results of this study reveal the relationship between the type of satisfaction of residents and subjective well-being. The study also provides answers to what can increase happiness after basic needs are met and suggests the direction of local government policies for community well-being.

Keywords Needs · Subjective well-being · Survey · Happiness

7.1 Introduction

Today, rapid changes in the environment demand changes throughout society. While the government was more faithful in its role as an exclusive supplier of public services, it was defined that the government is no longer an exclusive supplier of public services. Many of the services provided by the government or the public sector in the past have been transferred to the private sector and provided by market principles. People who used to be passive in government services have now started to voice their wishes for services. These changes eventually led to discussions regarding consumer-centered and customer-centered reforms in the public sector and public services sector. This change in the administrative paradigm requires the public sector to play a role in meeting the needs of consumers. Providing public services that meet the needs of individuals is the basic logic pursued by custom administration.

This is why it is more important for fundamental organizations that provide administrative services directly to the public to focus on the needs of local residents

Y. W. Kang · S. J. Lee (✉)
Graduate School of Public Administration, Seoul National University, 1 Gwanak-ro, Gwanak-gu, Seoul 151-742, South Korea
e-mail: slee@snu.ac.kr

Y. W. Kang
e-mail: oliviakang0120@gmail.com

© Springer Nature Switzerland AG 2019

Y. Kee et al. (eds.), *Perspectives on Community Well-Being*, Community Quality-of-Life and Well-Being, https://doi.org/10.1007/978-3-030-15115-7_7

so that actual customized service delivery is achieved. Basic organizations provide a variety of public services to local residents, such as roads, education, parks, water supply and drainage, and welfare for children, teenagers, and senior citizens. Thus, the ultimate purpose of local governments is to provide a variety of public services to their residents and to promote their welfare through the provision of public services (Lee, 1993).

From this point of view, if appropriate services are provided according to the needs of the residents, the welfare of the residents will be improved and happier. For this reason, it is important to discuss the needs of residents in research on the improvement of the well-being of residents through the provision of services.

As for individual needs, Maslow et al. (1970) seeks to achieve the desire of belonging as a social desire under the basic desire of survival desire and safety desire, and then seeks to pursue self-esteem desire. The important fact is that depending on the level of satisfaction of each of these needs, individuals have different needs. This means that there is a need for services depending on the level of satisfaction of residents. Therefore, what public service will affect the well-being of the residents after basic desires have been met?

Kahneman and Deaton (2010) suggested that after a certain income level, happiness would be affected by factors other than money. A study by Easterlin (1974) found that increases in income at the individual level of a country are closely linked to happiness, but not at the national level. In particular, in a society where basic living requirements are met, the increase in average income does not affect the average yield (Koo, Im, & Choi, 2014). However, this study has not been conducted.

The purpose of this study is to clarify the relationship between satisfaction type of residents' needs and subjective well-being. For this analysis, the organization conducts ranked logistic analysis using the 2017 Community Well-Being Survey of Korea. The results of this study reveal the relationship between the type of satisfaction of residents and subjective well-being. The study also provides answers to what can increase happiness after basic needs are met and suggests the direction of local government policies for community well-being.

7.2 Literature Review

7.2.1 Consumer-Oriented Administration and Residents' Needs

Public services are defined as the type of intangible goods and services government provides to the people. Services we receive from everyday life include buses, subways, pedestrian crossings, parks and libraries. These public services exist as administrative tools in order to achieve the purpose of increasing public welfare and improving national competitiveness. Lucy, Gilbert & Birkhead (1977) defined public services as the activities of the government that distribute benefits within society in order to create a desirable environment in society. Public services are the direct production, direct supply and delivery of goods, and services related to the benefits of the government to the residents. Goods or services are also produced by non-governmental entities such as interest groups, public corporations, and third-sector companies and are delivered to residents. Although public service is defined in various ways, the goods and services supplied to the society are called public services in order to increase the welfare and benefits of the residents in common. For the residents, public services are for the target of goods or services, which means that just like the consumer in the market, it is important for the consumer sector to understand what the consumer wants.

The consumer-centered administration regards the residents as users of services in the public sector as customers (Joo & Jung, 2000). This refers to efforts that enhance their welfare and benefits from the perspective of residents in order to improve their quality of life (Jeong & Park, 1999). Consumer-centered administration is an administrative system that emphasizes the residents who are more demanding than the government, which is the supplier, as to how and what service should be provided to improve the quality of life of the residents. Therefore, this study focuses on the satisfaction of the needs of residents and is important in the implementation of consumer-centered administration.

7.2.2 *Meeting the Needs of Residents and Subjective Well-Being*

The most classical way of explaining subjective well-being is the desire fulfillment theory (Diener, 1984). This means that subjective well-being (happiness and unhappiness) is determined by the fulfillment of needs. In this case, meeting various needs is proportional to environmental and situational conditions. Therefore, people with an environment that meets various needs are happier (Kwon, 2010). In other words, the environmental and situational conditions of the community in which the individual lives are the factors that influence the individual's subjective well-being.

This view is consistent with a study which showed that the level of subjective well-being did not always increase because of the well-equipped environmental requirements that satisfy basic needs (Peterson, 2006; Kwon, 2010). Conditions such as wealth, income, and status formed by education levels are negligible in relation to subjective well-being. For example, income level affects happiness beyond the level of poverty, but its impact is insignificant beyond that level. This is because money does not affect more than a certain level because money increases happiness through meeting basic needs (Veenhoven, 1991).

Before discussing how you can define the fulfillment of basic needs, we can look at the discussion of human needs. Maslow (1968) argues that humans have five basic needs as they live their lives, which have stages or sequences. The five needs include physiological needs, desires for safety, desires for belonging and love, demands for respect, and demands for self-realization. These five are classified into basic needs and upper needs according to their characteristics. The basic needs are met primarily by external factors, such as physiological needs, and safety and security needs. Growth needs are love and belonging, self-esteem, and self-actualization, and there are differences that are met by their internal factors.

Physiological needs are the basic needs of hunger, thirst, and warmth, which are the desire to be satisfied for survival. Sen (1987) refers to basic capability as a human being, such as food, clothing, shelter, and health, which is required to carry a minimum basic value. The lack of basic competence negatively affects the level of happiness. However, once basic competence is met, it is taken for granted and no longer acts as a positive factor in the satisfaction of life (Koo, Im, & Choi, 2014). In this way, it is reasonable to define the desire to pursue the things related to physiological desire, food and shelter, and to carry out the minimum thing as a human being is basic needs.

Safety is a fundamental desire of the basic element of human needs (Steers, Mowday, & Shapiro, 2004). The World Health Organization has declared the equal rights of health and safety as universal rights of all human beings (WHO, 1989) and the United Nations Development Program (UNDP) calls safety the essential condition of humanity and the sustainable development of a society (UNDP, 1994). In South Korea (hereafter, Korea), the collapse of the Mauna Resort in Gyeongju in February 2014, the Sungwol incident on the offing of Jindo in April 2014, and the fall of the Pangyo subway vent in October 2014 caused shocking disasters and safety accidents. These incidents became a top priority (Seo, 2015). No longer can security issues be solely accounted for by individual responsibility. Physiological needs and safety needs are basic needs and deficiencies such as hygiene factors (Herzberg, 1966), which do not have a positive effect on individual satisfaction levels but are negatively affected when they are deficient.

In this study, the desire for physiological needs and safety is defined as a basic desire, and the group of basic desires is satisfied. The importance of consumer-centered administration is increasing day by day. Nevertheless, it is difficult to find an empirical analysis of how public services provided by communities that form environmental and situational conditions, affect these groups. This study is different in that it considers the satisfaction of basic needs in discussing subjective well-being of an individual.

7.2.3 Subjective Well-Being and Public Service

Environmental and contextual conditions in communities affecting the subjective well-being of residents are shaped by the provision of public services. In this study, public services are divided into basic services, which provide benefits to a wide range of people according to their social functions and protective services, as development services provided by preference or selection of service subjects (Lucy, Gilbert, & Birkhead, 1977).

Routine services and protective services are comprised of basic public services. Routine services are commonly used by most people, including services such as water supply and drainage, roads and transport. These services may be limited to service use due to fees, and they are not purely public goods, as they may be personally provided.

Protective services are services that protect people and property and maintain public order, including security, police, and disaster protection. The performance of these services can be determined by the degree to which people are able to escape from the risks and harms through the service. However, these protective services require more care because the same police service and fire service alone cannot equalize the crime rate and fire rate in the jurisdiction.

Next, developmental services are services aimed at improving the physical, intellectual, and mental potential of individuals, and services such as education, libraries, parks, and consignment facilities belong to and are provided to almost everyone. This developmental service, however, has a distinctive feature for each individual in social functioning.

7.3 Analytical Data and Research Subjects

7.3.1 The Community Well-Being Survey

This study is based on the 2017 Community Well-being Survey. The Community Well-being Survey was conducted in Korea in 2013, 2015 and 2017. In 2013, out of five districts in Seoul, the districts selected for the survey were Guro-gu, Gangnam-gu, Dongdaemun-gu, Mapo-gu and Jung-gu, which represents each region based on the Median population. In the 35 questions, we examined the level of well-being in the community and the level of well-being in individuals. In 2015, the scope of the survey expanded to examine the well-being level of the individual and the well-being level of the community for adults aged 19 and over in 27 cities and counties across the country. The 2013 and 2015 surveys did not include satisfaction levels for individual needs. In 2017, a survey was conducted on how the five requirements of physiological needs, safety needs, belonging and affection, self-esteem, and self-fulfillment were satisfied. This research will use the 2017 survey.

The survey was conducted in November 2017 by the Community Well-Being Research Center of the Graduate School of Public Administration, Seoul National University, commissioned by Metrix Corporation. The participants in the questionnaire are adults aged 19 years and above who live in 27 cities and county districts of Korea. The sampling was a stratified random sampling approach, which was allocated proportionally by gender, age and region, with reference to the status of resident registration population as of September 2017. 100 respondents in each region answered the survey, and a total of 2,700 samples were collected. The response of the study participants consisted of a personal interview survey using a paper questionnaire. The purpose of the survey is to measure the level of community well-being in Korea and to search policy directions for community well-being. Therefore, the questionnaire is divided into 37 detailed questions about community well-being, and is divided into community evaluation items, questions about individual well-being level, subjective questions about satisfaction of individual needs, and socioeconomic characteristics of respondents.

7.3.2 *Characteristics of Respondents*

Respondents' characteristics were gender, age, educational attainment, income level, and relative income level, number of household members, residence period, socioeconomic status, marital status, and religion. First, about 50% are male, 20%, 20% and 30% are in their 20 s and 30 s, 40 s and 50 s, and 60 s, respectively. Second, as the age of respondents increases, the proportion of respondents increases, but the distribution is relatively even. Third, for educational attainment, 40% graduated from high school and from a two-year college. Fourth, one month's household income is divided by one million units. However, 264 people earned more than six million Korean won per month. On the other hand, 46.85 and 39.78% of the respondents said that their income is similar to those in the community and that their income is higher than the people around them, respectively. Fifth, 60 and 8% of the total number of household members is 3–4 persons and one person, respectively. Sixth, the percentage of married persons is as high as 76%. Eighth 1,740 people with a religion account for 64% of the total (Table 7.1).

7.3.3 *Subject of Study: Meeting Individual Needs*

In this study, we analyzed 2,700 respondents whose basic desires are satisfied. The 2,700 respondents were satisfied through their physiological needs (food, sleep, clothes, defecation, and sex life) and safety requirements (safe from physical, emotional and economic risks), and whether or not there is a difference between the two types of needs. This study divided physiological and safety needs into basic needs. Therefore, they responded to the demands of belonging (affection, friendship and love), self-esteem (self-confidence, achievement, honor and independence), and self-realization needs (self-development and potential exercise). In this study, two analyzes are conducted. Model 1 consists of 2,700 respondents, which is regarded as a whole group. And Model 2 analyzes the group in which basic needs are satisfied.

The survey was measured on a 10-point scale from very low (1) to very high (10) as to whether each of the needs were met. 7 or more points and below 6 points were classified as needs and unmet needs, respectively. Table 7.2 shows the number of responses for the lack of physiological needs and basic needs (safety requirements). 317 (11.7%) responded that their physiological needs were met but the safety requirements were not met. 263 (9.7%) responded that their desire for safety was met but their physiological needs were not satisfied. These two groups answered that one of the two needs was satisfied, but they were not all satisfied. Therefore, the respon-

Table 7.1 Statistical characteristics of respondents

Variable		Number	%
Gender	Male	1,361	50.41
	Female	1,339	49.59
Age	20–29	403	15.03
	30–39	414	15.44
	40–49	504	18.79
	50–59	537	20.02
	Over 60	824	30.72
Educational attainment	Middle school	494	18.30
	High school	1,144	42.37
	Over college	1,062	39.33
Monthly income level	Below 1,990,000	425	15.81
	2,000,000–2,990,000	441	16.40
	3,000,000–3,990,000	625	23.24
	4,000,000–4,990,000	540	20.08
	5,000,000–5,990,000	394	14.65
	Over 6,000,000	264	9.82
Relative income level	Not as high as others	361	13.37
	Similar to others	1,265	46.85
	Higher than others	1,074	39.78
Number of household members	1	217	8.05
	2	734	27.24
	3	695	25.79
	4	949	35.21
	Over 5	100	3.71
Residence period	Below 5 years	291	10.81
	5–9 years	357	13.27
	10–14 years	321	11.93
	15–19 years	239	8.88
	20–29 years	565	21.00
	30–39 years	352	13.08
	Over 40 years	566	21.03
Socioeconomic status	High within your area	378	14.03
	Middle within your area	2,212	82.08
	Low within your area	105	3.90
Marital status	Single	522	19.38
	Married	2,063	76.58
	Divorce, separation, bereavement	109	4.05
Religion	Yes	1,740	64.44
	No	960	35.56

Source The 2017 Community Well-being Survey of Korea

Table 7.2 Meeting basic needs

PPhysiological needs	Safety needs		
	Non-satisfaction	Satisfaction	Total
Non-satisfaction	411 (15.2%)	263 (9.7%)	674
Satisfaction	317 (11.7%)	1,709 (63.3%)	2,026
Total	728	1,972	2,700

Source The 2017 Community Well-being Survey of Korea

dents were not included in the basic needs fulfilling group. 1,709 (63.3%) respondents answered that their physiological and safety needs were all satisfied. In this study, we analyzed a total of 2,700 respondents and 1,709 respondents by basic needs.

Table 7.3 shows the demographic characteristics of those who answered that their basic needs were satisfied. First, the gender ratio for both males and females is close to 1:1 (50%). Second, the percentage of those aged 60 or older (27%) is slightly higher than those in their 40 and 50 s (20%) and 20 and 30 s (~16%). Third, 40.9% answered that their income was similar to those surrounding them, and 49.15% answered that their income was higher than those surrounding them. Fourth, 14–24% have monthly household income distributed evenly except for earning less than 2 million Korean won and over 6 million Korean won per month. Fifth, most respondents have 2, 3, or 4 household members, and the proportion of one person in the household (6%) is very low. Sixth, 20% responded that they stayed less than 30 years and 20% responded that they stayed more than 40 years in the residence area. Seventh, an overwhelmingly high response for "middle" socioeconomic status in the community was provided by the respondents. Eighth, 77% of the respondents are married.

7.3.4 Measurement of Variables

This study used exploratory factor analysis to measure the variables. First, we conducted an exploratory factor analysis to determine how many common factors account for 41 questions related to community well-being and individual well-being. As a result, three factors with 36 questions were extracted. The number of jobs in the area, the cost of living for local residents, the recycling and waste collection service, the cleanliness of alleys and streets, the degree of surrounding noise, and community well-being for public transport are not included in the three factors. All the questionnaires in this study were measured on a 10-point scale. Table 7.4 shows the factor loadings and reliability figures for each factor (Cronbach's alpha).

Table 7.3 Basic statistics of the research subjects

Variable		Number	%
Gender	Male	862	50.44
	Female	847	49.56
Age	20–29	266	15.67
	30–39	279	16.44
	40–49	331	19.51
	50–59	350	20.62
	Over 60	471	27.75
Educational attainment	Middle school	266	15.56
	High school	744	43.53
	Over college	699	40.90
Monthly income level	Below 1,990,000	192	11.29
	2,000,000–2,990,000	241	14.17
	3,000,000–3,990,000	408	23.99
	4,000,000–4,990,000	375	22.05
	5,000,000–5,990,000	285	16.75
	Over 6,000,000	200	11.76
Relative income level	Not as high as others	170	9.95
	Similar to others	699	40.9
	Higher than others	840	49.15
Number of household members	1	103	6.04
	2	450	26.39
	3	451	26.45
	4	641	37.6
	Over 5	60	3.52
Residence period	Below 5 years	189	11.08
	5–9 years	232	13.60
	10–14 years	196	11.49
	15–19 years	164	9.61
	20–29 years	368	21.57
	30–39 years	230	13.48
	Over 40 years	327	19.17
Socioeconomic status	High within your area	201	11.79
	Middle within your area	1,422	83.40
	Low within your area	82	4.81
Marital status	Single	333	19.54
	Married	1,321	77.52
	Divorce, separation, bereavement	50	2.93
Religion	Yes	1,078	63.08
	No	631	36.92

Source The 2017 Community Well-being Survey of Korea

Table 7.4 Exploratory factor analysis

	Questionnaire		Factor loadings		
	Number of Q	Contents	1	2	3
Basic public service alpha = 0.964	q1_6a	City/County/Administration	0.528		
	q1_7a	Degree of regional economic activation	0.509		
	q1_19a	Road maintenance level	0.549		
	q1_20a	Traffic level in the area	0.563		
	q1_21a	Pedestrian convenience	0.623		
	q1_22a	Disaster preparedness level	0.623		
	q1_23a	Police & Police Service	0.612		
	q1_24a	Health level	0.535		
	q1_25a	Medical Services	0.614		
	q1_26a	Elderly services	0.654		
	q1_27a	Disabled people services	0.660		
	q1_28a	Child care services	0.642		
	q1_29a	Participation in community organizations	0.647		
	q1_30a	Community's tenacity and collaboration	0.641		
	q1_31a	Trust in local residents	0.671		
	q1_32a	Trust in City Hall/County Office	0.734		
	q1_33a	Trust in the central government	0.681		
	q1_34a	Level of political information related to newspaper/TV	0.739		
	q1_35a	Fairness of public officials	0.756		
	q1_36a	Attitude and service of civil servants	0.763		
	q1_37a	Assessment of overall public services	0.793		
Developmental public services alpha = 0.902	q1_1a	Public library		0.542	
	q1_2a	Lifelong learning service		0.520	
	q1_3a	School level in the region		0.552	
	q1_4a	Living space (house)		0.527	
	q1_9a	Cultural activity level		0.552	
	q1_10a	Local cultural facilities		0.534	
	q1_11a	Local tradition/culture/value		0.538	
	q1_13a	Air pollution degree		0.509	

(continued)

Table 7.4 (continued)

	Questionnaire		Factor loadings		
	Number of Q	Contents	1	2	3
	q1_14a	Parks and green spaces		0.591	
	q1_15a	Water quality of rivers/lakes/oceans in the region		0.609	
Subjective well-being of individual dimension alpha = 0.889	q2_1	Overall life in the area			0.897
	q4_1	The engaged life			0.673
	q4_2	The meaningful life			0.552
	q4_3	The pleasant life			0.642

Source The 2017 Community Well-being Survey of Korea

7.4 Research Design

Ordered logistic regression analysis was conducted to analyze the relationship between subjective well-being and public service in the individual dimension of the group whose basic needs were satisfied. Subjective well-being (dependent variable) at the individual level was measured on a 10-point scale in sequence. In this case, since it is not possible to use general linear regression analysis or ordinary least squares (OLS) estimation, the model used in this study is the ordered logistic regression model. Ordered logistic regression analysis is suitable for measuring the effect of independent variables on ordered dependent variables. In order to measure the subjective well-being of the individual dimension the questionnaire survey was conducted on the overall life: the pleasant life, the engaged life and the meaningful life at the individual level.

First, a 10-point scale (1 = very low, 10 = very high) was measured for overall life in the area. The 10-point scale measures to eliminate the central tendency of respondents for the variables. The degree of empathy for each of the three statements '(1) I am satisfied with my life', '(2) My life is meaningful', and '(3) My life is good' was measured on a 10-point scale (1 = not at all sympathetic, 10 = very sympathetic). The dependent variable used the mean score for the above four items to measure the subjective well-being at the individual level.

The independent variables in this study were measured by an assessment of the level of community related to basic public services and by an assessment of the level of communities involved in the development of public services. Questions related to basic public services were measured on a 10-point scale (1 = very low, 10 = very high) for the local economy, infrastructure and health, and welfare and local administration services. Survey items related to basic public services include the disaster preparedness level, policing and police services, health level, medical services, elderly services, disabled services, and childcare services. The items related to developmental public services are related to the local education, culture, and environmental services, such as public library, lifelong education service, cultural activity level, air pollution level, and are measured on a 10-point scale (1 = very low, 10 = very high).

The demographic variables used as control variables are gender, age, educational attainment, income level, and relative income level, number of household members, tenure, socioeconomic status, marital status, and religious status. Because they pursue social status rather than income itself, relative income levels as compared to the others can influence individual well-being and thus are reflected as a control variable (Clark & Oswald, 1996). Marriage is important for subjective well-being. In the cases of separation, it is said that the level of subjective well-being is lower than in the cases of divorce or bereavement (Helliwell, 2003). Religion was reflected as a control variable as religious people easily overcome difficulties in life (Frey & Stutzer, 2002).

The characteristics of the dependent and independent variables considered in this study and the measurement of the variables are summarized below in Table 7.5.

Descriptive statistics describing the attributes of each variable are shown in Table 7.6. The subjective well-being of the individual dimension, the dependent variable, is the average of 1709 people whose basic desire is satisfied (7.55). In the case of the group in which the basic needs were satisfied, the average of community well-being evaluations for basic public services and developmental public services as independent variables was 6.94 and 7.05, respectively.

7.4.1 Research Model

This study derives a research model composed of basic public services, developmental public services, and subjective well-being at the individual level as shown in Fig. 7.1. Basic public services and developmental public services in the region lead to the improvement of subjective well-being at the individual level according to the upward diffusion theory. The reason for this is that according to the upward diffusion theory (Sirgy & Su, 2000; Sirgy et al., 2008), the perception of an individual's well-being is formed through comprehensive utility in each life domain. Thus, this study uses the results of an assessment of basic public services and advanced public services in the region in which respondents reside, as well as the results of a survey on individual life. On the other hand, the function of public service affects individual needs differently. Therefore, this study suggests the necessity of verifying according to the function of the service through the satisfaction data of the individual's life according to the degree of satisfaction of the individual's needs.

The hypothesis (H) assume the relationship between public service and basic needs, and individual well-being. Regardless of the type of service provided in the region, the higher the level of public service provision, the higher the subjective well-being of individuals. H1 and H2 are as follows.

H1 The higher the level of basic public services provided in the region, the higher the subjective well-being of the whole group.

Table 7.5 Measurement of variables

	Variable	Name	Measure
Dependent variable	Subjective well-being of individual dimension	Overall life in the area, The engaged life, The meaningful life, The pleasant life	Average of responses to each questionnaire
Independent variables	Basic public services	City/County/Administration, Degree of regional economic activation, Road maintenance level/Traffic level in the area pedestrian convenience, Disaster preparedness level, Police & Police Service, Health level, Medical Services, Elderly services, Disabled people services, Child care services, Participation in community organizations, The community's tenacity and collaboration, Trust in local residents, Trust in City Hall/County Office, Trust in the central government, Level of political information related to newspaper/TV, Fairness of public officials, Attitude and service of civil servants, Assessment of overall public services	Average assessment at the community level for each survey (1 = very low, 10 = very high)
	Developmental services	Public library, Lifelong learning service, School level in the region, Living space (house), Cultural activity level, Local cultural facilities, Local tradition/culture/value, Air pollution degree, Parks and green spaces, Water quality in rivers/lakes/oceans in the region	Average assessment of the level of community for each survey (1 = very low, 10 = very high)
Control variables	Gender	Male = 1, Female = 0	
	Age	20–29 = 1, 30–39 = 2, 40–49 = 3, 50–59 = 4, Over 60 = 5	
	Educational attainment	Middle School = 1, High School = 2, College = 3	
	Monthly income level	A month's pre-tax household income (Below 1,990,000 = 1, Over 60,000,000 = 6; Scale of one million won)	

(continued)

Table 7.5 (continued)

	Variable	Name	Measure
	Relative income level	Not as high as others = 1, Similar to others = 2, Higher than others = 3	
	Number of household members	One person = 1, 2 people = 2, 3 people = 3, 4 people = 4, Over 5 people = 5	
	Residence period	Below 5 years = 1, 5–9 years = 2, 10–14 years = 3, 15–19 years = 4, 20–29 years = 5, 30–39 years = 6, Over 40 years = 7	
	Socioeconomic status	Low within your area = 1, Middle within your area = 2, High within your area = 3	
	Marital status	Single = 1, Married = 2, Divorce, Separation, Bereavement = 3	
	Religion	Yes = 1, No = 2	

Source The 2017 Community Well-being Survey of Korea

Table 7.6 Descriptive statistics of the variables

	Variable	Observation	Mean	S.D.	Minimum	Maximum
Dependent variable	Subjective well-being of individual dimension	1,709	7.55	0.81	3.75	10.00
Independent variables	Basic public services	1,535	6.94	1.02	2.86	9.86
	Developmental services	1,666	7.05	0.95	3.30	9.50
Control variables	Gender	1,709	0.50	0.50	0	1
	Age	1,697	3.28	1.42	1	5
	Educational attainment	1,709	2.25	0.71	1	3
	Monthly income level	1,701	3.54	1.50	1	6
	Relative income level	1,709	2.39	0.66	1	3
	Number of household members	1,705	3.06	1.01	1	5
	Residence period	1,706	4.34	2.01	1	7
	Socioeconomic status	1,705	1.93	0.40	1	3
	Marital status	1,704	1.83	0.44	1	3
	Religion	1,709	0.37	0.48	0	1

Source The 2017 Community Well-being Survey of Korea

H2 The higher the level of developmental public services provided in the region, the higher the subjective well-being of the whole group

In addition, changes in the level of public services provided in the region will have different impacts on the groups for which basic needs are met. H3 and H4 are as follows.

H3 The effect size of basic public services will be relatively low as compared to the general individual.

H4 The effect size of developmental public services will be relatively higher for individuals with basic needs fulfillment than those for general individuals

Table 7.7 shows the subjective well-being of respondents by demographic variables.

7.5 Results

This study estimated the effects of the characteristics of basic public services and developmental public services on the subjective well-being of the individual under the control of demographic and sociological characteristics. The subjective well-being of the individual, which is a dependent variable of this study, was measured by a 10-point scale in which the order existed, and a rank-based regression analysis was conducted to examine the effect of the explanatory variables on the dependent variables. The results of the analysis are shown in Table 7.8. Model 1 is an analysis of the entire response to the questionnaire. Model 2 is intended for groups that have responded to basic needs.

The results of the analysis of Model 1 (whole group) show that basic public services (0.623) and developmental public services (0.342), which are public services provided by the community, have a statistical significance of 0.1%. The odds ratio, which indicates the proportion of individuals' subjective well-being increase for the whole group, was estimated to be 86.4 and 40.7% for basic public services and developing public services, respectively. This means that as the level of basic public service evaluation provided by the community increases, the overall well-being of individuals increases by 86.4%. As the level of developmental public services increases, the subjective well-being at the individual level can increase by 40.7%. The income level and the relative income level in the whole group have a positive effect on the subjective well-being of the individual at a significance level of 0.1%.

Socioeconomic status and residence period also have a positive effect on the subjective well-being of individuals at the 5% significance level. The number of household members, religion, and educational attainment have a negative impact on individual subjective well-being at the 0.1, 1, and 5% significance level. In addition, gender, age, and marital status were not statistically significant, indicating that they did not significantly affect individual well-being.

In Model 2 (satisfying basic needs), regression coefficients for the evaluation of basic public services and developmental public services of the community were

Table 7.7 Subjective well-being at the individual level by demographic variables

Variable		Observation	Mean	SD	Minimum	Maximum
Gender	Male	862	7.53	0.84	3.8	10.0
	Female	847	7.56	0.78	4.0	9.5
Age	20–29	266	7.56	0.83	4.5	10.0
	30–39	279	7.50	0.75	4.5	9.8
	40–49	331	7.56	0.82	4.5	9.5
	50–59	350	7.57	0.84	3.8	10.0
	Over 60	471	7.53	0.81	5.3	10.0
Educational attainment	Middle school	266	7.59	0.85	5.5	10.0
	High school	744	7.52	0.83	3.8	10.0
	College	699	7.56	0.78	4.0	9.5
Monthly income level	Below 1,990,000	192	7.56	0.90	4.8	10.0
	2,000,000–2,990,000	241	7.41	0.83	5.0	9.3
	3,000,000–3,990,000	408	7.49	0.85	3.8	9.5
	4,000,000–4,990,000	375	7.67	0.76	5.0	8.8
	5,000,000–5,990,000	285	7.58	0.74	5.0	9.3
	Over 6,000,000	200	7.52	0.79	4.0	9.8
Relative income level	Not as high as others	170	7.24	0.96	5.0	10.0
	Similar to others	699	7.38	0.84	4.0	10.0
	Higher than others	840	7.75	0.70	3.8	10.0
Number of household members	1	103	7.50	0.92	4.5	10.0
	2	450	7.63	0.82	5.5	10.0
	3	451	7.59	0.75	5.0	9.0
	4	641	7.47	0.81	3.8	9.3
	Over 5	60	7.48	0.99	5.3	9.5
Residence period	Below 5 years	189	7.33	0.88	4.8	10.0
	5–9 years	232	7.51	0.76	4.0	9.0
	10–14 years	196	7.50	0.72	5.3	8.8
	15–19 years	164	7.56	0.77	5.3	9.0
	20–29 years	368	7.59	0.80	4.5	9.8
	30–39 years	230	7.63	0.81	4.5	10.0
	Over 40 years	327	7.62	0.87	3.8	10.0
Socioeconomic status	High within your area	201	7.34	0.79	4.8	10.0
	Middle within your area	1,422	7.56	0.81	3.8	10.0
	Low within your area	82	7.74	0.81	5.5	9.3
Marital status	Single	333	7.54	0.83	4.5	10.0
	Married	1,321	7.54	0.81	3.8	10.0
	Divorce, separation, bereavement	50	7.57	0.80	5.5	10.0
Religion	Yes	1,078	7.55	0.82	4.0	10.0
	No	631	7.54	0.80	3.8	10.0

Source The 2017 Community Well-being Survey of Korea

Table 7.8 Ordered logit regression results

	Model 1 (all)			Model 2 (basic needs satisfaction)		
	β	Std. error	OR[a]	β	Std. error	OR
Basic public services	0.623***	0.056	1.864	0.394***	0.078	1.484
Developmental public services	0.342***	0.059	1.407	0.377***	0.083	1.458
Gender	−0.0912	0.073	0.913	−0.068	0.093	0.935
Age	−0.0353	0.040	0.965	−0.042	0.052	0.959
Educational attainment	−0.173*	0.067	0.841	−0.041	0.089	0.960
Monthly income level	0.124***	0.031	1.132	−0.020	0.041	0.980
Relative income level	0.540***	0.065	1.716	0.544***	0.081	1.722
Number of household members	−0.172***	0.042	0.842	−0.165**	0.056	0.848
Residence period	0.0474*	0.021	1.049	0.116***	0.027	1.123
Socioeconomic status	0.217*	0.096	1.242	0.0976	0.121	1.103
Marital status	0.0523	0.106	1.054	−0.031	0.138	0.970
Religion	−0.202**	0.076	0.817	−0.242*	0.097	0.785
No. of observations	2,445			1,505		
Log likelihood	−6481.7043			−3677.074		
Chi^2	1021.97			328.94		

* $p < 0.05$, ** $p < 0.01$, *** $p < 0.001$
[a]OR = odds ratio

0.394 and 0.377, respectively, showing a positive effect on individual subjective well-being at a level of 0.1%. In the group responding that basic needs were met, both types of public services also show that they are affecting subjective well-being. The relative income level, which is the income level in comparison to other people in the community and the residence time in the community, are 0.1% statistically significant, indicating a positive influence on the subjective well-being of the individual. The number of household members and religion shows a negative (−) effect on subjective well-being at the 1 and 5% significance level. Unlike the whole group, income level, socioeconomic status and education level were not statistically significant in the groups where basic needs were satisfied.

The analysis of the two models discussed above provides meaningful conclusions. The factors influencing the subjective well-being of individuals in the model separate the entire group of respondents and the groups whose met basic desires are discriminatory.

Next, we will look at similarities and differences in the relationship between the two groups and different types of public services. First, in a similar way, both groups that meet the basic needs and the entire group have positive relationships between the assessment level of basic public services in the community and the subjective well-being of individuals. This supports H1. In the case of developmental public services, the result of a positive relationship in both groups supports H2. The results of this statistical analysis can be assumed that the higher the level of public service provision, regardless of the type of service provided by the local community, the more positive the impact on subjective well-being at the individual level. On the other hand, the same results in the two groups are different from general predictions. Maslow argues that after basic needs are met, people seek the next step. Herzberg and Sen argue that basic needs no longer influence well-being once basic needs are met. For this reason, additional research is needed to see if the level of basic public services affects the group in which basic needs are satisfied. In this study, those who responded with 7, 8, 9, or 10 on a 10-point scale were selected for the group in which basic needs were satisfied. This is because there is a limit to the fact that the basic needs are fully satisfied and the needs of the next stage are needed. Second, we will look at the differences between the two groups and the types of public services. In both groups, the effects of public services are positive, but the degree of meaning in each group is different. In the case of the whole group, the difference between basic public services and developmental public services is larger than the basic needs fulfillment group. The odds ratios were 1.864 and 1.407 for the whole group, and 1.484 and 1.458 for the basic needs group. These results suggest that it is difficult to support the hypothesis that changes in the level of public services provided in the region will have a different impact on the group in which basic needs are satisfied. Specifically, individuals in the basic needs group do not support the relatively high magnitude of developmental public services effect than the general individuals in H4. On the other hand, a further study is needed in the sense that the effect of basic public services will be relatively low in the individuals who meet a basic desire than the general individual in H3. Although the whole group shows that the impact of basic public services is greater than the developmental public service impacts, it does not support the small effect of basic public services in the basic needs fulfillment group. These results show that basic public services are important to everyone and are still a field that should not be overlooked even if the needs for physiological needs and safety are met.

Now, we look at similarities and differences in the sociocultural aspects of the two groups. First, the similarities are statistically significant in both groups: relative income, duration of residence, number of households, and religion. In the community, the higher the level of their income as compared to the others, the longer the period of stay in the area, the more positive the effect of subjective well-being. On the other hand, the higher the number of households, the less negative effect on subjective well-being. Second, the difference in the demographic and sociological aspects of the two groups was found to be significant only in the whole group, including income level, educational attainment, and socioeconomic status. In the basic desire satisfaction group, the income level was not statistically significant but showed subjective well-being and negative direction. However, in the whole group, the higher the income level was, the statistically significant effect of a positive influence on subjective well-being was verified at 0.1% level.

7.6 Conclusion

The source of public service demand is the needs of local residents. The difference between the demand level of the residents and the demand level that is currently achieved, can be defined as 'demand for public services'. Therefore, in order to improve the quality of public services, local governments must first recognize the needs of the residents and determine what to deliver and how to deliver.

The purpose of this study is to classify services provided at the community well-being level as basic public services and developmental public services. We tried to present the direction of a well-being community in order to implement a consumer-centered administration. The results of the study suggest some important points that the government should consider in presenting the direction of a well-being community.

First, basic public services are important to everyone. In other words, basic desire is satisfied for the group of residents or the whole group confirmed that basic public services positively affects the subjective well-being. These results imply that a basic public service provision is still important, even when the needs for physiological needs and safety are met. Basic public services are required for a group whose basic needs are not satisfied, and a group already fulfilled does not mean that basic public services are unnecessary. Therefore, it is necessary to study basic services by subdividing basic services to see what types of services have more influence on subjective well-being. Furthermore, it is necessary to understand what policy or budget allocation contributes more to the subjective well-being of the community's inhabitants. This implies that the local government's provision of public services needs a more thorough evaluation of the causal path leading to the establishment of a well-being community and the improvement of subjective well-being of residents.

Second, developmental public services have a relatively greater impact on satisfaction with the type of needs satisfaction. According to the results of the study, both the whole group and the group whose basic desire is satisfied, have a greater impact on basic services. However, the effect of basic services and developmental services is large in the whole group, but the effect of the two services is small in the group in which the basic desire is satisfied. The impact of basic public services is significantly greater in the whole group, but it is not so after the basic needs have been met. In the present study, it was concluded that the results were not satisfied because the physiological needs and safety needs were not completely satisfied. Therefore, it is necessary to closely examine the impact of developmental public services on subjective well-being through a study that distinguishes groups that satisfy basic needs completely.

To implement a consumer-centered administration, services are selectively provided to specific groups such as children, the elderly, and women. It is necessary to provide differentiated services by distinguishing the degree of satisfaction of the desire within the specific object as well as the specificity of the object. If the demand level of the consumer is differentiated and the supply of differentiated services is provided properly, improvement of personal well-being through the promotion of community well-being will also be a shortcut. Despite the policy implications, there are limitations of this study. In the research methodology, the results of the single-year survey in 2017 were analyzed. Therefore, it will be necessary to study the needs of the residents who change according to the point of view through continuous research and time-series data collection.

Acknowledgements This work was supported by the National Research Foundation of Korea Grant funded by the Korean Government (NRF-2016S1A3A2924563).

References

Clark, A. E., & Oswald, A. J. (1996). Satisfaction and comparison income. *Journal of Public Economics, 61*(3), 359–381.

Diener, E. (1984). Subjective well-being. *Psychological Bulletin, 95*(3), 542.

Easterlin, R. A. (1974). Does economic growth improve the human lot? Some empirical evidence. In *Nations and households in economic growth* (pp. 89–125).

Frey, B. S., & Stutzer, A. (2002). What can economists learn from happiness research? *Journal of Economic Literature, 40*(2), 402–435.

Helliwell, J. F. (2003). How's life? Combining individual and national variables to explain subjective well-being. *Economic Modelling, 20*(2), 331–360.

Herzberg, F. I. (1966). *Work and the nature of man*. Oxford, England: World.

Jeong, Y. S., & Park, K. H. (1999). An analysis of the customer orientation of the local government information service. *Korean Journal of Policy Analysis and Evaluation, 9,* 85–103.

Joo, J. H., & Jung, Y. S. (2000). Policy suggestions for the establishment of the public service charter program. *Korean Public Administration Review, 34*(1), 245–264.

Kahneman, D., & Deaton, A. (2010). High income improves evaluation of life but not emotional well-being. *Proceedings of the National Academy of Sciences, 107*(38), 16489–16493.

Koo, K. J., Im, J. Y., & Choi, S. G. (2014). Determinants of happiness: Reevaluating the role of income and capability. *Korean Public Administration Review, 48*(2), 317–339.

Kwon, S. M. (2010). The relation between desire and happiness from the viewpoint of psychology. http://s-space.snu.ac.kr/bitstream/10371/68751/1/v.36_121.pdf.

Lee, S. J. (1993). A balanced analysis of public service distribution in local government. *Korean Association for Policy Studies, 2*(1), 188–206.

Lucy, W. H., Gilbert, D., & Birkhead, G. S. (1977). Equity in local service distribution. *Public Administration Review,* 687–697.

Maslow, A. H. (1968). Some educational implications of the humanistic psychologies. *Harvard Educational Review, 38*(4), 685–696.

Maslow, A. H., Frager, R., Fadiman, J., McReynolds, C., & Cox, R. (1970). *Motivation and personality* (Vol. 2). New York: Harper & Row.

Peterson, C. (2006). *A primer in positive psychology*. Oxford: University Press.

Sen, A. (1987). *Gender and cooperative conflicts (No. 1342)*. Helsinki: Wider.
Seo, J. H. (2015). An Exploratory Study on the Safety Needs as a Motivation of Citizen's Safe Behavior : Based on Maslow's Hierarchy Theory of 5 Basic Needs. *Korean review of crisis and emergency management, 11*(6): 207–225.
Sirgy, M. J., & Su, C. (2000). Destination image, self-congruity, and travel behavior: Toward an integrative model. *Journal of Travel Research, 38*(4), 340–352.
Sirgy, M. J., Gao, T., & Young, R. F. (2008). How does residents' satisfaction with community services influence quality of life (QOL) outcomes? *Applied Research in Quality of Life, 3*(2), 81.
Steers, R. M., Mowday, R. T., & Shapiro, D. L. (2004). The future of work motivation theory. *Academy of Management review, 29*(3), 379–387.
Veenhoven, R. (1991). Is happiness relative? *Social Indicators Research, 24*(1), 1–34.

Young Woong Kang is a research fellow at the Center for Well-being Research at the Korean Institute of Public Affairs, Seoul National University, Seoul, South Korea. In August 2017, Korea University received a Doctoral degree in Public Administration (dissertation title: A study on the Institutional condition of Public Service Delivery by Market Mechanism: focusing on the Elderly Care Service Voucher). Areas of interest include public service delivery, institutional analysis, collaborative public management, and policy analysis. In her book, there is a case study on people who are dreaming of a society without corruption (2011, co-author). In recent articles, "A Study on the Status and Role of the Autonomous Management Fishing Community: A Legal Perspective" (2018), "The Formation Process of the Autonomous Management System in Korea: Autonomous Management Fishing Policy" 2016).

Seung Jong Lee is a Professor and Dean of the Graduate School of Public Administration, Seoul National University. Previously, he served as the president of the Korean Association for Public Administration and as chief editor of several academic journals in related fields. He has frequently advised local and national governments through such positions as chairman of the Local Government Administration Joint Evaluation Committee, vice-chairman of the Presidential Committee on Local District Reorganization Plans, and member of the presidential transition committee. He has not only done extensive research on citizen participation and local autonomy but has also been a strong advocate and educator in the field. He is the author of *Theories of Local Autonomy,* and *Democratic Politics and Citizen Participation.*

Chapter 8
Shredding the Evidence: Whose Collective Impact are We Talking About?

Geoffrey Woolcock

Abstract There has been considerable hype in Australia recently accompanying the North American-informed Collective Impact (CI) approach and its claims to deliver real transformative social change for individuals and communities. CI actively promotes its principal incentive and distinctive trait, namely to concentrate the energies of its collaborators to achieve real, long-term, measurable and sustainable outcomes, often quoted as a Social Return on Investment (SRoI). Not coincidentally, the rise of CI's visibility has emerged alongside diminishing public funding for social change initiatives, with a corresponding and somewhat belated turn to the philanthropic sector to partially meet this funding shortfall. Early signs across Australia indicate that philanthropic funds are no less driven by a 'value for money' imperative than governments that in turn, has left many lamenting the shift in community organisations working to satisfy donor expectations rather than working with and for local communities. In this context, some serious questions have already been raised about the Collective Impact approach and ambition, particularly how CI can meaningfully engage with long-term disadvantaged local communities and realistically agree on what successful outcomes would look like for such communities. Community cultural development (CCD) would seem to offer a useful counterpoint to the CI approach with its enduring emphasis on authentic process and bottom-up solutions but CCD too has received its own share of criticism for an obsession with process to the exclusion of real and tangible social outcomes. Whatever approach's claims are to be tested, this paper starts from the standpoint that their veracity will only be significant if they can actually demonstrate they are making a difference in our most disadvantaged communities and populations.

Keywords Collective impact · Measuring well-being · Community cultural development · Community indicators

G. Woolcock (✉)
Institute for Resilient Regions, University of Southern Queensland, Queensland, Springfield/Toowoomba, MA 4350, Australia
e-mail: Geoffrey.Woolcock@usq.edu.au

© Springer Nature Switzerland AG 2019

Y. Kee et al. (eds.), *Perspectives on Community Well-Being*, Community Quality-of-Life and Well-Being, https://doi.org/10.1007/978-3-030-15115-7_8

8.1 Introduction

The Maven Project of the community arts organisation *Beyond Empathy* (BE) in regional Northern New South Wales, Australia is a three-year project (2014–2016) that builds an Aboriginal community arts and cultural development hub using a process which first engages, then works collaboratively on planning and creatively developing. The genuine CCD process that Maven engages in is already producing demonstrable outcomes but not those that are traditionally valued and counted in social change initiatives. Focusing on Maven and BE, this paper sets out to challenge all those who purport to support outcome-oriented social change approaches to more thoroughly assess the process by which outcome measures are proposed and then agreed upon. It thus seeks to demonstrate the fundamental connection between CCD and social change outcomes and measurement, a connection that would seem to be somewhat tangential for many purveyors of Collective Impact (CI). Furthermore, it also seeks to challenge those seeking to revive CCD approaches to not only engage in but develop a more sophisticated outcomes and measurement vocabulary and help turn around the distorted but commonly held perception that CCD is disinterested in quantification of outcomes.

8.2 Beyond Empathy

Beyond Empathy (BE) is a community, arts and cultural development organisation that "uses the arts to influence change in the lives of individuals and communities experiencing recurring hardship".[1] It works in regional areas across Australia seeking to break cycles of disadvantage and help individuals to develop new skills.

Beyond Empathy's stated purpose is to:

- Use art to influence real change and enhance the well-being of the lives of marginalized individuals and communities.
- Give the most disadvantaged people in society opportunities to participate in, and create vibrant, innovative and culturally ambitious works of art.
- Create extraordinary art and through that, develop the skills and tools people and communities need (confidence, reliance, self-worth, self-knowledge) to succeed beyond anyone's expectations.
- Generate new connections and new opportunities overriding disengagement and disadvantage.
- Go further than any other organisation, to places no one else goes; delving into situations no one else will touch; reaching people no one else can reach; collaborating with everyone, rejecting no one.

BE's diverse history of CCD is well recognised for achieving positive relationships and results with marginalised communities, particularly regional and remote

[1] From Beyond Empathy's webpage, www.be.org.au.

Aboriginal communities. BE operates with a strengths-based approach and the overarching principle of partnership over paternalism; and, participation over theory. Emerging artists across all art forms are provided an opportunity to build capacity, foster experimentation and develop original work in collaboration with professional artists. For some of BE's participants, this process has led to sustainable employment. The Maven project alone created 15 arts employment opportunities, allowing for ongoing employment pathways, while 63 emerging artist dance, music, song, poetry/written word, production, photography, intensive workshops were held with 12 emerging artists.

More recently, BE has engaged external evaluation consultants in some of its larger projects where initial results demonstrate measurable health and social improvements, particularly a SRoI study conducted by NetBalance of BE's *Rites of Passage* film project that showed for each dollar invested, a social return of three times that amount was delivered through improved emotional well-being, increased self-esteem, improved prospect of meaningful employment, improved outlook for the future, increased social inclusion & improvement in personal relationships.

This focus on impact is articulated by BE as aiming "to create a benchmark model for measuring our social impact and mirroring our CCD leadership" through implementing an "arts led social impact strategy" based on a Logic model/approach, alongside other measurement concepts. The rationale is that "[l]ogic models are a logical or systematic way to articulate and share understanding about the relationship between what is invested (money, people, expertise) + activities (what we do) + outputs (people served, things created) + outcomes (changes that happened in people or community) resulting in IMPACT – long terms changes in people, policy or practice directly attributable to Beyond Empathy's work".

Perhaps as equally significant as BE's ten principles[2] guiding its work with community, is BE's stated eight values guiding its *social impact measurement*, namely:

- Take responsibility for impact and encourage others to do so too.
- Focus on our purpose.
- Involve others in our impact practice.
- Apply proportionate and appropriate methods and resources.
- Consider the full range of the difference we make: positive and negative, planned and unplanned.
- Be honest and open.
- Be willing to change and act on what we find.
- Actively share our impact plans, methods, findings and learning.

Furthermore, BE measures its artistic vibrancy against six parameters:

- Reflection—did it move you?
- Aesthetic merit—was it well put together and was the art product of a high standard?
- Delivery—was it well put together and well presented?

[2]http://10principles.be.org.au/.

- Experience—did it introduce you to new experiences or opportunities, things you've not encountered before?
- Insight—did it introduce you to new thoughts, did you learn new things?
- Reflection—did you think about people differently?

There is plentiful evidence that BE has 'walked the talk' in terms of applying these principles and parameters in its innovative Maven project. As an umbrella for a number of specific initiatives—including 3 Moree, Catharsis, Festival of the Brolga and Festival of the Brave, and emerging artists' intensives—Maven has demanded that all the principles and values underpinning its delivery have been strongly tested.

8.3 Maven

The Maven Project is a three-year project commencing in 2014 that builds an Aboriginal community arts and cultural development hub in Armidale, NSW. The Maven project uses a process which first engages, then works collaboratively on planning and creatively developing. The process is always about gathering together as a collective. Aboriginal autonomy and ownership sits at the centre of the Maven Project. Part of the need for the Project is the ongoing socio-economic disadvantage that characterises the area with Armidale, Moree and the surrounding region of north-west NSW having lower levels of income and higher levels of unemployment than the national average. The region has below average educational participation and incomes and a large Aboriginal population comprising 5.8% of Armidale's population and 22.8% of Moree's population, compared with the state average of 1.9% (about 10% of the NSW Aboriginal population live in the region), and they experience unemployment rates as high as 46%.

Educational disadvantage is higher in the region with 69.6% of women and 61.4% of men having no skilled post-school qualifications (compared with State averages of 65.2 and 53%). The weekly income for a single person is 17% below the national figure and the weekly income for a household is 21% below the national figure. The percentage of one-parent families in the region is 20.3%, which is over 30% higher than the national average of 15.5%.[3]

With low levels of educational attainment and high unemployment rates, the Aboriginal young people in North-West NSW require projects that engage them with the community on several levels—with their culture, with elders, with local support services and with different skills training not solely reliant on the traditional manual trades qualifications. Proposed projects must recognise Aboriginal young people's strong connection to culture and their inherent talent in the arts.

The Maven Project respects the deep cultural cycle of life-long learning and teaching that guide Aboriginal communities and recognizes that Aboriginal people

[3]Data drawn from NSW Office of Aboriginal Affairs (2018) *Community Portrait of Moree, accessed at* https://www.aboriginalaffairs.nsw.gov.au/new-knowledge/facts-and-figures/community-portraits.

have all they need to teach and guide their young people and their communities to artistic and cultural independence. Unique to Maven is the creation of enabling spaces for Aboriginal people and artists to take the lead with their skills, with support and backing from BE building their leadership in a sound and supportive cultural context where they set the rules of engagement. By continually adapting and molding projects around them and their skills, each experience cascades into the next, but only when they are ready. Such a process sometimes jars with Collective Impact approaches reliant on large systems where partners can rarely be this flexible, most notably education, bound by timetables and rigid rules that mitigate risk and disruption, in direct contrast to BE's belief that it is in the chaos that learning occurs and creativity develops.

Mavens are intense gatherers of information and impressions and so recognise that art and narrative sits at the centre of all teaching and learning. Driving the Maven Project are the Aboriginal teachers, mentors and cultural guides necessary to take their community into the next millennium. Mavens are information-hoarders and information brokers, sharing and trading what they know.

The Maven Project sought to create a hub for creativity, imagination, collaboration, learning, skills, cultural exchange and community development in Armidale, NSW using the development of two major cross-artform performance works and the exceptional artistic and cultural talents of professional Aboriginal artists as the platform to grow the creative hub. Working as artistic leaders and teachers, they used the opportunity to participate in two annual major cross-artform performance works to unlock the potential of young emerging Aboriginal artists from across regional NSW who have untapped strengths. Maven placed Aboriginal artists at the centre of the creation of a major artistic work with their community about their community. It is a hallmark of the project's approach to give Aboriginal people full custodianship over their intellectual property, to be in charge of how their work is created and how they present it to the broader community.

Such a committed approach can have significant implications and most certainly did in Armidale where Maven's institutional partners found it very difficult to relinquish this custodianship over creative intellectual property when the "crunch" of performance time arrived. While a collaborative approach had certainly acknowledged the input of these institutional partners in co-creating performance spaces, ultimately a lack of genuine support for the performers themselves and the intent of the final community outcome resulted in poor audience numbers at the annual event and in turn, saw Maven take the lion's share of the blame as the visible performers being assessed against perceived outcomes. For BE's Executive Director, a collective impact approach "means for us that there are too many variables to control and too many things can go wrong at the last minute and ultimately, that's bad for the participants—who need to benefit most from the big-bang final outcome. Then the creative team is judged rather than the systems people because people expect artists to be unwieldy but the truth is they have greater pride in their work than any other professional".[4]

[4]Via email from BE Exec Director, February 2015.

The Maven project also placed young people at the centre of its activity, recognising that they are the future and sustainability of Aboriginal communities wanting to be valued and seen as contributors to their community, but needing new opportunities to prove themselves. Now in its third year, *No Shame Day*—showcasing remarkable and inspiring performances by young people sharing positive youth culture, reflecting on personal experiences, and creating performance works that acknowledge their capacity to influence their future—has been championed by BE as precisely one of these new opportunities. A similar motivation underpinned photographer Raphaella Rosella's Admire exhibition where Moree East children were asked 'If you had one wish, what would it be?' and the richness of the responses created opportunities for perceptions to be challenged through the beauty of the works produced.

Knowing the arts and creativity are such powerful tools to enable this change, the Maven Project provides the space for young people to be aspirational; to be taught and mentored by highly acclaimed Aboriginal artists who have succeeded against all odds becomes living proof that with new options (provided through the creative hub) and with increased opportunities, disadvantage doesn't have to dictate one's future. Additionally, the Maven Project develops arts and culture in the New England and Northwest region, creating a hub for excellence where professional Aboriginal artists work across many art genres including music, dance, physical theatre, film and design to create a major artistic work with young people and community to reimagine their future. This provides a creative framework for young emerging Aboriginal artists where they develop professional skills, collaborate, co-create and present new works to audiences. By working alongside these artists, they develop confidence, experience and skills to develop their careers as artists and as Mavens. Through Maven, significant new artistic projects were developed including the Divine writing and subsequent theatre project developed with Cathy Craigie in Armidale and Mnemonic developed by Kirk Page for contemporary dance/body work/performance project to work with BE emerging dance artists.

8.4 Catharsis

One of the more prominent and visible initiatives of the Maven project to date has been *Catharsis*. A paper shredding machine was set up in a pop up shop's front window in Armidale's main street for the public to participate in the cathartic process of writing and then shredding their thoughts and feelings until the space fills with discarded emotions, anxieties and tensions. The installation and the CCD process surrounding it sought to alleviate stress, anger, hopelessness and sadness, and leading ultimately to emotional relief. Poems and word sculptures came to life on the window as the background filled with shredded paper. After the shredding, BE invited the participants to contribute words and thoughts that reflect their unencumbered state of mind, their aspirations, affirmations and dreams for the future. These were recorded by either or all of three methods: (i) interview on a laptop, (ii) writing on the shop's wall or (iii) in a post it box. The Catharsis space was open for four weeks in mid-

2014. These recorded words and affirmations were also used to compose two songs, under the tutelage of prominent indigenous and local artists, and a play with a local writer.

What emerged from the Catharsis workshops was that young people palpably identify they have few prospects. They believe they have been failed by the education system, rarely have jobs, have babies early because they want to be loved, are often "open cases" with government because boyfriends use the Department as a threat and have few chances of being regarded for the distinctive individuals they are. Further stages for Catharsis through the final months of 2014 included paper-making workshops at the New England Regional Art Museum (NERAM), the production of three video documentaries at NERAM involving projections onto recycled paper made from the pop-up shreddings, installation of vinyl text affirmations to be displayed in CBD shop windows, and finally an exhibition at NERAM.

From various artists that were in residence at Catharsis, the great positive is that the process is so simple and thus is easy to garner good participation across all demographics, especially age, race and education. There was a significant response from people dealing with personal problems right through to people who live with mental health issues, scribed by one of the residing artists:

> Isabel, who has bipolar, visited many times. On her first visits, she just scribbled in an expressionist manner on five or so pieces of paper. She would remain about an hour, and then shredded. On her sixth visit, she brought in many pieces of thin black cardboard with tracings already drawn. She proceeded to cut them out, revealing black clouds, her symbol for depression. In addition, she cut out eight differing shapes of houses. Isabel has issues in cleaning and emptying out all her housing investment real estate. She procrastinates so long that issues such as these are not addressed, acted upon or solved. This only further compounds her situation. Her houses remain unleased. Isabel is blessed with being a great artist but has no self confidence in herself. The cut-out houses confirmed her original artistic talent. I took a photo of her works before they were shredded.

Catharsis was an important contributor to the overall Maven Project with a total of 467 participants coming into the pop-up shop over the four-week period of its installation. When this paper's author asked one of the residing artists what evidence of impact he would cite for what is going on at Catharsis, he shot back "Right there in front of you, that pile of shredded paper!" It is worth noting that sometimes initiatives like Catharsis are designed explicitly for private healing and not for assessment purpose and true community engagement respects this. While this approach might seem counter to one that is open to all processes of engagement being subject to rigorous scrutiny, an alternative viewpoint is that grounded community cultural development needs to stand strong on retaining privacy so that communities can genuinely trust a CCD process unlike the trust that has been eroded over the years through so many pilot programs inflicted on marginalised populations and communities.

8.5 3 Moree

The 3 Moree program, with the support of local Aboriginal Education Consultative Group and the Moree East public school community, offered a continuum of learning and support initially through connecting with parents and caregivers in antenatal stages, supporting transition into early childhood learning and then foundation years through to stage 3 outcomes of primary education. Through the use of arts, a safety net was created to ensure all families are involved.

3 Moree had three components:

- Mubali—an innovative health intervention strategy using creative art processes as a bridging tool to connect young Aboriginal Women (14–24 years old) to local Aboriginal midwifery services and generalist health services;
- Connexion—working with 0–8 year old children, their families and the existing Schools for Community program to improve connection to early childhood opportunities, knowledge and learning;
- Festival of the Brolga—alignment to the curriculum, one-on-one mentoring and arts led workshops, produced the Festival of the Brolga, an annual community festival that celebrates identity and drives connections between the school, the community, families and culture. The project worked closely with local elders and other community members in the school to tell the story of the Brolga (a native waterbird) and its relevance to modern day Moree. The project was based around workshops with young people, developing their technical and story-telling skills in dance, performance, theatre, film and song. The content and inspiration for these workshops came from the elders' and community stories and their living memories.

What emerged in the evaluation of 3 Moree was the ongoing resistance of established systems of health and education to creative interventions that empowered marginalized people, young and old, to become genuinely involved. An email exchange towards the conclusion of the 'Admire' initiative (involving young students led by an emerging BE artist) between the resident school authority and BE is poignantly illustrative of these tensions:

School authority:

Hi [BE staff]

The handwritten story by [young student] needs to be edited.

Get her to hand write it again (same blurb) but use capital A for Aboriginal and change the word 'won' to 'one'.

Then it is OK with me.

Reply

BE staff:

Hi [School Authority],

I'm sorry, I can't change the portrait. The text is an extension of [young student]'s portrait and identity and it would be unethical to correct it. The portraits belong to the creators (the children and [indigenous artist]) and they are not for us to change.

In this instance, I think we could safely say these beautiful children are teaching us what it is to be human.

Have a good day,

Reply

School authority:

My call. [young student] will need to edit it as this is all part of the writing process and [young student]has not had the opportunity to do this.

The upshot of this firm and authoritative stance for CI approaches is that while the intent of the NSW Education Department's *Connected Communities Strategy* is laudable and aligned with CI theory/approaches, its translation is so dependent on creative and flexible leadership that was quite evidently lacking here.

What is also at play is that school educators are clearly being driven by performance outcomes over and above those for the most affected students where fear rules in being perceived to have achieved satisfactory traditional academic performance benchmarks.

If culture, creativity and inventiveness has the ability to change outcomes for Aboriginal children and their families and as valued by their community, but is met with resistance from the system that has 'committed' to doing business differently, the challenge is to know what teachers would need to feel competent in genuinely moving to a more creative approach or way or working?

For BE's Executive Director, they need to "reposition themselves as learners". Just how difficult this is when most teachers are increasingly inundated with reporting to mostly irrelevant traditional performance indicators and outcomes has been highlighted by Maven and BE, whose approach demands BE are learners because ownership of the BE process is handed over to community and BE follows their lead. As BE's ED explains, "we learn from community what the next step is and in the creative processes, the making of art becomes the response. The language of creativity becomes a common language and builds the roadmap for each step in the journey. We are space creators; our role is to enable the space for community to be the teachers. We listen, we learn and we try to implement with community what they want to see happen for their community and for their children. It is often unruly, disruptive and it's loaded with chaos. The process is not linear and at times we all experience a feeling of groundlessness when we have no idea where it's all going. We expect to make honest mistakes. The nurturing of warm, real relationships (the disorderly type ones that exist in every family) are the foundation. And indeed Carl Jung says it is this warmth that is vital for the growing plant and the soul of the child." [5]

Of course, it should be emphasised that such a process need not eschew outcome indicators and consistent with the commitment to impact assessment outlined above, BE have already managed to cite multiple successful outcomes from the Maven Project including results not cited earlier:

- Quantitative and qualitative data demonstrated significant improvements in participant self-efficacy and capacity to influence their future;

[5] ibid.

- Artistic practices were led by community with results demonstrating increased cohesion across community and with relationships with school. Over 90% of parents believe BE programs can improve school attendance, strengthen identity and help learning compared to 25% of teachers.
- 75% parents indicate BE programs strengthen pride in culture compared to 25% of teachers.
- 78% indicate BE programs strengthen relationships between children and community compared to 25% of teachers who think only somewhat and 25% not at all. 2303 page views on website since October of which 67.85% are new visitors;
- 5 conference presentations undertaken;
- Artists articulate benefits of The Maven Project as
  - ownership over work;
  - developing new skills;
  - support to work on new ideas; and
  - provision of artistic control and creative independence.
- Three artists develop new works to undertake with support of BE; and
- Two artists working on new creative ideas.

8.6 CCD and Social Change Outcomes

Renowned indigenous playwright and director Wesley Enoch's provocative (2014) essay *Take Me to Your Leader—The Dilemma of Cultural Leadership* amongst plenty of goading to the arts community, cries out "Did we ever have a purpose in our communities? Did you? Have we just forgotten it? Misplaced our meaning for a short time? Are we waiting for our brilliance to be finally recognised and for us to be rewarded by the masses without ever talking to them?"

This author's response to Enoch's plea in relation to indigenous community cultural development is to posit that there has never been more of an imperative to directly link measurable indigenous well-being outcomes with indigenous CCD practice. BE talks "with the masses" routinely and Maven is clearly a manifestation of the response to these conversations, but it nonetheless remans difficult to say precisely where BE is going or what will be achieved because its activity evolves from the conversations with community, whilst being governed always by their ten principles—that is consistently the anchor. While it is well understood that Aboriginal and Torres Strait Island arts are amongst the oldest art traditions in the world and art has always been an important part of indigenous life, actual measures remain limited to indigenous participation in indigenous cultural activities and perceptions of indigenous arts. Certainly, measures such as the 2014 *Arts in Daily Life: Australian Participation in the Arts* reporting 92% of Australians believing that 'Indigenous arts are an important part of Australia's culture', may indicate the continuing vitality of indigenous cultural heritage and wide participation as a significant means of maintaining group membership and cultural identity, but the achievements remain acknowledged almost entirely within the arts and cultural sector. Recognition of the importance of indigenous arts extends further to laudable federal government funded initiatives such as the Indigenous Cultural Support (ICS) projects including an objective to "promote Aboriginal and Torres Strait Islander well-being by strengthening pride in identity and culture" but again there is little onus placed on linking with measurable well-being outcomes for indigenous communities. To be clear, this is not to suggest that artistic professional development programs ought to have their funding tied directly to the achievement of improved well-being measures but rather to encourage the large scale social change and collective impact initiatives targeting indigenous communities to more actively integrate CCD into their implementation and assessment. How does, for example, an evaluation capture the feeling of the raucous 600 strong audiences cheering their kids on when it is so difficult to survey them on the spot, and audio-visual material sadly remains a poor substitute for rigorous evidence?

The most pertinent Australian example in this respect would undoubtedly be the Closing the Gap initiative. Interestingly, the 2013 Closing the Gap commissioned discussion paper *Engaging with Indigenous Australia* while observing that Aboriginal and Torres Strait Islander peoples and communities know and articulate the many benefits of keeping culture strong, "the evidence base lags behind community voices and experiences as the effect of culture is difficult to measure. However, there is a growing body of research supporting the community view that positive outcomes stem from keeping culture strong". Hunt (2013), in summarising 'What we don't know' (p. 4), further emphasises missing evidence across a number of scenarios:

- We don't know how to overcome the persistent challenges governments face in trying to engage on the ground in a flexible, whole-of-government way within systems that are based on upward departmental accountabilities;
- It isn't known how to engage effectively where an Indigenous community is in conflict, has highly fractured governance or has weak leadership;
- There is little or no research evidence about successful engagement arrangements in urban areas or the Torres Strait Islands;
- There is no research evidence about either models of engagement for national or other levels of policy development or the role of Indigenous peak bodies in engagement strategies;
- The evidence from the most recent innovations by various jurisdictions in relation to engagement models and approaches is not available;
- The range of sectors for which there is significant research on successful approaches to program/project level engagement is limited;
- Research evidence of how free, prior and informed consent has been put into practice in governmental engagement processes and its impact is not yet available.

For all the significant work that was undertaken to create the six Council of Australian Governments (COAG) Closing the Gap targets,[6] it must not go unrecognised that scant attention has been given to how community cultural development

[6]Close the life expectancy gap within a generation.
Halve the gap in mortality rates for Indigenous children under five within a decade.

processes might be an effective mechanism to actually achieve these targets. As it happens, a number of initiatives associated with *Closing the Gap* have engaged the arts and cultural sector but the perception is more one of an accidental than a deliberate engagement with the arts. At least some of the missing evidence, or what we *don't* know cited above, may well lie in BE's cultural performances, exhibits and audience responses (e.g. shredded paper) permeating through indigenous CCD processes but not articulated in the traditional language of research and evaluation outcomes. It might also lie in the CCD processes that BE commits to where they can confidently cite plentiful examples of responses that indicate they do know many of the answers to Hunt's (2013)'what we don't know' dot points above.

8.7 CCD and Collective Impact

Of course, it has not gone unnoticed that in the emerging professional field of cultural development, funders and host organisations increasingly seek to understand the impact of work they support or lead. Arts and cultural sector leaders are challenged in this environment to fully explicate outcomes. Evaluation approaches infrequently take a holistic approach, instead often focusing predominantly on social or economic outcomes. Commonly, other outcomes are sometimes categorized as *intrinsic* and therefore considered immeasurable. Consequently, as Dunphy notes in her new co-edited book *Making Culture Count: the Politics of Cultural Measurement,* "much of the benefit of arts engagement can be missed… evaluation approaches commonly only consider benefits, and offer no assessment of negative or neutral outcomes, or proportion of benefit to costs". This is definitely a trap that BE has diligently sought to address, asking honest questions of itself and partners in identifying why certain initiatives were more effective than others, and not only upon reflection but dynamically during the lifecycle of a project like Maven.

Dunphy proposed a solution to those dilemmas via a holistic framework for evaluation of outcomes of arts engagement. The framework pre-supposes an intention by program leaders and funders to make a positive contribution to the lives of participants, and in so doing, to the wider community. It is proposed as useful for government (national, state and local), non-government and community organisations as well as individual artists and arts workers who have a positive change goal and seek to understand the implications of their work. The framework offers a means of considering different: *perspectives* of change (who perceived and experienced the change); *dimensions* of change (what type of change occurred); and *degree* of change (how much change occurred), to arrive at an overall assessment of project outcomes.

Halve the gap for Indigenous students in reading, writing and numeracy within a decade.

Halve the gap in employment outcomes between Indigenous and non-Indigenous Australians within a decade.

Within five years, all four year olds in remote Indigenous communities have access to quality early childhood education programs.

At least halve the gap for Indigenous students in Year 12 or equivalent rates by 2015.

Taking this holistic approach, it was apparent in 3 Moree that significantly different perceptions of change and effectiveness between the teachers and the community emerged and any authentic evaluation framework must be prepared to grapple with these differences.

But however holistic the perspective on change, if it is only to assess outcomes of a particular project—even a very large project—the impact is still likely to be relatively contained and highly context dependent. Here emerges the promise of Collective Impact (CI) with its challenge to the traditional model of a community group identifying an isolated need, then creating a service for that need, demonstrating results, and scaling their service to more people in hopes of creating larger societal change. CI instead begins with changing the community overall and works backward. It begins by setting a goal (for example, any of the COAG Closing the Gap targets) and then builds an ecosystem of nonprofits, government agencies, schools, businesses, philanthropists, local community groups and community leaders who create common strategies and coordinate integrated activities among them to achieve the goal.

The highly credible community activist Paul Schmitz and a regular commentator on collective impact has identified a few concerns about how CI gets implemented in a seminal piece *The Real Challenge for Collective Impact* (Huffington Post, 2012). Firstly, he identifies that the process by which leaders from different organizations, sectors, and levels of influence come together for CI is incredibly important and should not be rushed. These efforts, if done well, will require dedicated engagement, patience, deliberation, debate, and conflict. Secondly, he worries that the relentless focus on short-term data can trap groups into doing the most measurable activities, not necessarily the right ones. Members of CI efforts may remain focused on isolated needs and outcomes rather than thinking in a more integrated way about problems and long-term solutions. Thirdly, to solve our social problems in our communities, Schmitz suggests the solution must be to build stronger communities, not just stronger programs and services and yet, many CI efforts are still all about institutions and organizations doing things *to* communities, not *with* communities. In this context, CCD entities like BE that are so fundamentally committed to working closely with communities become even more important in an environment promoting collective impact. My own experiences to date of CI initiatives in Australia is that while there is a strong commitment to community development processes, the CI core principle of "shared measurement" is still largely left to university-based researchers to both determine and implement, flying in the face of letting the community itself gauge what is reasonable social return on investment.

Perhaps Schmitz's most telling observation is that while much of the early research and work on collective impact has emphasized the structural, strategic, and measurable, "to succeed long-term, there must be more attention paid to the cultural. Culture is created through shared values, expectations, and goals. These must be built intentionally, transparently, and evolve with the project". How early CI initiatives in Australia might face up to this considerable challenge—including the incorporation of community cultural development practice into a framework so focussed on measurable outcomes—is already looming as one of the 'game-changing' moments for CI and its authenticity, particularly in indigenous communities. To this end, BE has legitimate claims as a "game changer" because this is how it works, with BE expecting things to get worse before they get better, hence demanding that sufficient *time* is required.

8.8 Measuring (Cultural) Progress

Another significant intersection faced by the growing interest in community cultural development measurement and impact is its relationship with the citizen-based global progress measurement movement which has emerged in the past decade, with its potential for realisation of a new paradigm for democracy, good governance and authentic cultural engagement. The benefits emerging already from this movement appear to be significant. These include new and more dynamic forms of democratic engagement; the demonstration of clearer linkages between strong democratic and human rights regimes, and broader individual and societal well-being; new ways to define and measure a 'healthy' democracy; and perhaps most importantly, a re-examination of the nature of progress and democracy in the 21st century. The limited extent to which cultural indicators have featured in the emergence of the global progress measurement movement and its democratising ambitions is revealing and whilst it is a reminder of a long way to go, Woolcock and Davern's (2015) 'Creative Accounts' chapter demonstrates that there are significant place-based community indicator systems like Community Indicators Victoria (CIV) that stoke some optimism.

CIV aims to improve the community well-being of all Victorians by creating equitable, engaged, healthy and well-planned communities through evidence based policy and planning, reporting and monitoring, and enhanced democracy. The indicator system forms an important resource for local governments in Victoria following amendment of the *Public Health and Well-being Act 2008 (Vic.)* which stipulated the use of evidence for deciding on health priorities and interventions during municipal public health and well-being planning based on a four year planning cycle. One area of health and well-being of particular interest to local governments and communities is the importance and value of the arts. Very limited data exists on the use and measured impact of the arts on community well-being, despite a widely acknowledged acceptance of the social and economic benefits to the wider community. Very few quantitative sources are available as evidence of this value despite estimates of cultural and creative activity contributing $86 billion to Australia's national accounts in 2008–2009.

Arts and culture were included in the CIV framework of community well-being in recognition of the importance of these activities for community identity and the role of art, film and literature for interpretative communication on contemporary social issues. Early consultation in the development of the framework suggested the inclusion of arts and culture indicators that measured *actual participation* in arts and cultural activities as well as *opportunities for participation* in arts and cultural activities. The focus on participation provided a narrow measure of the arts. This is consistent with the role of community indicators, which are not designed as all-encompassing measures. Indicators are effectively the tip of the iceberg and act as a monitoring tool, providing a starting point for further investigation and community discussion. Indicators are, by definition, aggregated data or broad measures of community progress that need to be anchored to policy levers to create future change. They also need to measure issues deemed important to a community (as identified in the consultation process leading to the development of the CIV framework), monitor trends and drive advocacy or action for future change. With a growing list of indicators included in the CIV framework, the arts indicators included in CIV were designed as broad measures that could be understood by the general public in a large scale community survey. Most importantly, *opportunities to participate* in arts activity in the local area were separated from actual *participation* to measure local access, and general community support that might not translate into individual interest or actual involvement. CIV is a unique and rare provider of indicator data on arts participation and opportunities for arts participation but as its coordinator Melanie Davern writes in a chapter of MacDowall et al's (2015) edited volume on community cultural develepoment measurement, "future indicators of arts should aspire to expand beyond participation and focus more on the diverse contribution of art in creating healthy, cohesive and engaged communities". Again, there is plenty of evidence gathered by BE—albeit not in the form of traditional quantitative indicators—that puts forward a compelling case for its significant contribution to creating more healthy, cohesive and engaged communities. The more such evidence can be incorporated into larger regional progress indicator initiatives, the more confident we can all be that these are indicators of genuine progress.

8.9 Conclusion

Certainly, the scale at which community-driven progress and sustainability indicators have grown in the past decade suggests that what began as a series of diverse experiments is already a global movement. And there is now some optimism that this global movement may bring a paradigm shift in public policy, which threatens to replace two long dominant assumptions: the primacy of continuous economic growth as the key driver of well-being; and the historically powerful but deterministic notion of the 'inevitability of progress'.

In their place, this new paradigm offers a more holistic, integrated and nuanced model that recognises the interdependence of economic, social, cultural, environmental and democratic dimensions for equitable and sustainable well-being: that is, genuine progress. The most important outcome of the OECD's project on measuring progress may ultimately be the fact that it has launched a global democratic debate about the meaning of progress.

This conclusion was strikingly evident in November 2007 for anyone attending both the European Union conference 'Beyond GDP' in the European Parliament in Brussels, and immediately after, the Third Gross National Happiness conference in Chang Mai, Thailand. The language and values were different, and the settings and participants could not have been more dissimilar, but the message from both of these very different conferences was exactly the same: 'It is time to end the mismeasurement of progress by economic growth alone, and to move to a new and more legitimate paradigm that is people centred, equitably distributed and environmentally and socially sustainable'.[7]

How community cultural and artistic measures of progress integrate with the broader global movement still remains uncertain, particularly in the face of many neo-liberal western governments determined to return to narrowly struck economic growth agendas in the shadow of the global financial crisis and another potentially looming. The CIV example, however, is illustrative of how bottom-up community indicator initiatives can enable a genuinely democratic approach to measures of progress, an endeavour that is critically reliant on the arts and cultural sector to contribute integrated measures.

As both the Australian Cultural Minister's Council (2011) *Vital Signs: Cultural Indicators for Australia* and Australia Council (2014) *Arts in Daily Life* papers demonstrated, there is visible recognition that measuring the value of culture and art is becoming increasingly significant, but the challenge of determining the most effective measures and at various scales stubbornly persists. As the Chair of the National Cultural Policy Reference Group, Julianne Schultz (2013) observed at the *Arts and Public Life Breakfast Series* in Sydney:

> We have to be more ambitious and smarter in finding a way to measure the public value of culture. We know it exists, but we have not yet found the right way to measure it. We also have to be more ambitious in measuring the intrinsic value of the work produced by artists and the costs that fall disproportionately on them and their families because their work is not properly valued; the institutional in terms of a national ethos which draws visitors or inspires productive innovation; the instrumental value, like the well documented legacy for children of exposure and involvement in arts and culture to successful and engaged lives, and the commercial value which is contributing more to the national economy than many other sectors.

We could do a lot worse than to kick-start this collective ambition to better measure culture's value with a solid grounding in community cultural development and practice that not only unashamedly prioritises local community's outcomes but just as importantly, actively engages the community in determining the way these outcome measures should be constructed and then attained. So, in short, beyond empathy....

Acknowledgements This work was supported by the National Research Foundation of Korea Grant, funded by the Korean Government (NRF-2013S1A3A2054622), and the CCD organisation, Beyond Empathy.

---

[7] As articulated in UNDP (1996, p. iii).

References

Australia Council. (2014). *Arts in daily life: Australian participation in the arts*. Sydney: Australia Council.

Cultural Ministers Council. (2011). *Vital signs: Cultural indicators for Australia* (1st ed.). Canberra: CMC Statistics Working Group.

Enoch, W. (2014). *Take me to your leader: The Dilemma of cultural leadership* (Currency House, Platform Papers No. 40).

Hunt, J. (2013). *Engaging with indigenous Australia: Exploring the conditions for effective relationships with aboriginal and torres strait islander communities* (Australian Institute of Health & Welfare, Closing the Gap Clearinghouse Issues Paper No. 5).

MacDowall, L., Badham, M., Blomkamp, E., & Dunphy, K. (Eds.). (2015). *Making culture count: The politics of cultural measurement*. Melbourne: Palgrave.

Schmitz, P. (2012). The real challenge for collective impact. *Huffington Post*. Retrieved February 7, 2015, from http://www.huffingtonpost.com/paul-schmitz/collective-impact_b_1920466.html?ir=Australia.

Schultz, J. (2013, August 14). Where to from here…after the National Cultural Policy. In *Arts & public life breakfast series*, Sydney. Accessed through subsciption at Currency House Platform Papers, https://currencyhouse.org.au/node/264).

United Nations Development Programme (UNDP). (1996). *Human development report 1996* (p. iii). Oxford: Oxford University Press for UNDP.

Woolcock, G., Davern, M. (2015). In L. MacDowall, M. Badham, E. Blomkamp, K. Dunphy (Eds.), *Making culture count: The politics of cultural measurement*. Melbourne: Palgrave, pp.129–144.

Geoffrey Woolcock is a Senior Research Fellow at the University of Southern Queensland's Institute for Resilient Regions an Adjunct Associate Professor, Griffith University's School of Human Services and Social Work. He works with a diverse range of public and private sector organizations helping develop whole of community outcome measures for a variety of social interventions, particularly in socio-economically disadvantaged communities. He is especially interested in building more effective evidence of which place-based approaches work to improve community well-being.

Chapter 9
Fiscal Structure and Residents' Well-Being in Korea

Youngkyun Oh

Abstract Local financial expenditures have been the subject of focused inspection in Korea. There is little research devoted specifically either to the self-accountability of local governments or to a residents-oriented expenditure system. This chapter, in the context of local financial accountability, is an effort to find a way to reorganize the role apportionment for community well-being and explore it from the fiscal structure perspective.

Keywords Fiscal dimensions · Subjective well-being

9.1 Introduction

What are some of the most issues facing societies today? In this chapter, the focus is on one of these, the well-being of community residents and relationships between local governance of financial resources and allocation. In South Korea (hereafter, Korea), two financial subjects have been institutionalized after the restoration of local self-governance in the efforts towards democratization and localization. There has been a continuing debate over if the financial double structure system is an effective mean to promote the efficiency and competitiveness of a country. Similarly, in Korea, there are issues on overlapping investments and wasteful local programs. If we approach this by dichotomous thinking, the central point of contention is how to distribute a country's limited financial resources between the central and local governments for national growth. However, the local view is how to increase the residents' well-being. While the central government's interventions in local financial affairs has increased, the autonomy of the financial operations of low level governments has decreased. Laying out a system of reasonable standards for the relationship between the central and local governments is by no means an easy task. The central government can establish rules for the programs of local governments and can

Y. Oh (✉)
Dean of Humanities & Social Science College, Suwon University, Seoul kangnamgu dokog street 242 samho apt. 1-1105, Gyeonggi, South Korea
e-mail: oyk241@daum.net

© Springer Nature Switzerland AG 2019

Y. Kee et al. (eds.), *Perspectives on Community Well-Being*, Community Quality-of-Life and Well-Being, https://doi.org/10.1007/978-3-030-15115-7_9

offer some revenue sources. In this way, the local discretionary scope became narrow and residents became less responsible. Since the second half of the 1980s, with the revival of local self-governance, the Ministry of Government Administration and Home Affairs of Korea has expanded their legal basis and guiding principles for strengthening managerial functions. In particular, the system of inspection of local financial expenditure was considered as a special object for focused inspection. From the 1990s, there has been a trend for the governments to establish new structures of inter-governmental relationship and to set up local financial accountability. Within the area of financial restructuring, some distinction is defined between revenue and expenditure. However, concerning the systems of proper role allocation, there is little research devoted specifically either to the self-accountability of local governments or to a residents-oriented expenditure system. This chapter, in the context of local financial accountability, is an effort to find a way to reorganize the role apportionment for community well-being.

For a long time, debates concerning the efficient use of financial resources have been tending towards the strengthening of centralized control. However, there have also been lively arguments for increasing financial accountability of local governments. Some of the theories such as the internalization of the external effect and the alleviation of information asymmetry may be useful for us to understand the confused situation.

9.2 Theoretical Debate

If one considers a close look at the results of previous research focusing on the decisive factors for expenses in Korea, it seems the factors that show a local government's financial capability like the fiscal self-reliance ratio, the gross regional domestic product (GRDP) and the financial independence ratio, cannot explain the variation of local expenses. Lee and Dong (2007) claim that the greater transfer from higher government, the greater social welfare expenses for local self-governing bodies. This means that local self-governing bodies determine the welfare expenses according to the fiscal budgets of the central government. Choi (2008) analyzed the financial growth of local self-governing bodies in terms of income, industrialization, the number of civil servants, government funding and the previous year's expenses. The results of this analysis showed that income tax, population size, number of civil servants and previous year's expenses partly explain the finances of a self-governing body. Kim and Hong (2011) analyzed subsidy rates, structure of parties and welfare budget level variables. Their research results show that financial autonomy has a negative effect on social welfare costs per person. Lee et al. (2005) set their dependent variables as child care budget and adolescent budget scale. They set their independent variables as rate of financial autonomy, rate of budget increase, rate of budget decrease, and the party to which the community head belongs. This research shows that financial autonomy and rates of budget variation have a positive effect. Also, according to the type of region, the party to which the head of the local government belongs, the number of people living in basic security within the local autonomous government have a positive effect. Many studies show that the indicator of local taxes per person is statistically insignificant. The most relevant research in terms of content and method is that of Soh (1998). This study analyzes the effects of changes in the welfare system to a self-governing body. Soh (1998) simply compared wealthy self-governing bodies to weak self-governing bodies instead of using a regression analysis of all basic self-governing bodies. In particular, we can consider structural change models for social welfare expenditures and non-social welfare expenditures and compare tax revenue ratios to welfare expenditures in autonomous districts.

The local autonomous budget factors can be divided into social, political and financial factors. The social factors include the basic living guarantee recipient rate, senior population rate, disabled rate and adolescent child rate. The political factors include belonging to the party of the head of local government, population rate, whether or not there is a local election and the type of local autonomous self-government. The financial factors include the rate of financial autonomy and the amount of local taxes. So far, social factors have been regarded as insignificant because welfare costs are a small portion of the economy and have a tendency to grow according with the number of welfare recipients. The higher the number of welfare recipients, the more effect on a local region. The financial factor is affected by the local autonomous government's capacity. This includes the financial autonomy rate, financial index and local taxes per person. The most widely used index of financial autonomy is the difference in ratio of local tax revenue and non-tax revenue of the total tax revenue. This represents how independent the autonomous governing body is. The financial independence ratio expresses how much of a local government budget is from independent revenue sources (i.e., local grants taxes, adjustment grants and subsidies) and is a useful indicator for figuring out how much financial resources can be mobilized by themselves. However, previous research shows that the higher the rate of fiscal autonomy, the lower the level of welfare finance. This means that there are other factors to explain the welfare expenses. Thus, we should review the political-economic aspects simultaneously.

9.3 Political-Economic Aspects

Non-social welfare estimates such as economic development and general administration budget are also related with the budget. When the input becomes bigger, the averaged fixed cost becomes smaller. Thus, through average cost shrinking, in comparison to an urban area, the possibility for an increase in the average unit production expense for welfare services in a small rural population region is high. In this way, there are alternatives of which indicators we should use. In many cases, the needs in estimates of residents' welfare is negatively correlated with the budget itself at the community level. However, the total quantity of demand affected the social welfare budget estimate. The welfare budget was especially positively correlated not with their real demands but the number of recipients receiving the basic living security.

Thus, we can guess that this is due to the impacts of basic living security guarantee estimates and there is a positive correlation between people who receive the basic living security guarantee, and the size of the social welfare budget needs.

Historically, a subsidy was a means for the central government to control local governments.

The scale of the central government's subsidy expands local autonomy and local accountability becomes weaker. In Korea, the central government's basic welfare system is based on the central government nationwide public programs. Due to the separateness of the central intentions and local executive system for welfare, the moral hazard of the principle-agent relationship can be a significant problem. The requirements of financial information on the progress of the subsidy projects of regional self-governing bodies leads to significant information asymmetry. Actually, the central government is unable to assess their progress and performance without the correct response of local governments and agencies. From the perspective of self-governing bodies, the funds of the central government are just another public asset. The enticements of the central government's resources leading to competition among regional self-governing bodies may cause the political prisoner's dilemma at any time.

9.4 New Public Management

In order to understand the role allocation and competition among governments, we need to consider new public management (NPM) as a theoretical background. NPM tries to achieve better results by strengthening autonomy and accountability. Thus, new public management emphasizes empowerment and performance of local governments. NPM is similar to market federalism in that it adopts market elements that stress the competitiveness for providing high quality public service. NPM also suggests a horizontal contract system not only within a government but also among governments. In this context, NPM prefers to strengthen local autonomy and accountability. However, NPM differs in that it was introduced as a governmental reform theory for dealing rapidly changing external factors, unlimited competition, severe cutbacks and government distrust. Thus, NPM emphasizes an overall framework established through a downward orientation in order to improve strategical performance. In order to develop a performance framework, a practical way is to equip competition methods, and while in the process of execution, the voluntary participation of relevant organizations is emphasized. More than their approaches to political economy, the biggest difference is outcome-oriented program management and governmental reform. Peter Drucker's results management and decentralization or perhaps the Osborne Geblar's 'Reinventing Government' belong here. With regards to mid-level systems management, this comes close to Tiebout and Oates' governmental financial relations and other similar microscopic approaches of Neo-classical political economy.

New public management emphasizes result orientation and central government leading to promote governmental reform. The integration of a vision, goals, strategy, action and feedback management-related central government mechanism for planning and the drafting of an annual performance plan are all required. According to the central government, the individual regional financial groups are integrated within the central government's separate ministries and offices. Within individual vertical management systems, regional finances are absorbed into the lower departments of the central government. For business effectiveness and economy, businesses need to be managed effectively. Following this, in the central government, guarantee and verification of the needed outcome information, a management system is established, and extensive knowledge is necessary. In consideration to the intended results of governmental reform, we can see the appropriateness of a local transfer of functions. Following this, on the basis of adding public cooperation values, the applicability of the principle is limited. If the central government's performance budgeting based on a program become stronger, local government's accountability and autonomy become weaker. In that situation, local competition can be emphasized without consideration of the community well-being of residents.

9.5 Policy Issues

9.5.1 Decentralization and Accountability

Historically, the actions of regional civil servants are criticized and recognized that the vertical financial managerial supervision of the central government is needed. On the other hand, efforts to build regional civil society and responsibly cooperative financial governance are sorely needed. The capacities of managerial supervision over regional financial operations has grown stronger, while the regional financial efficiency and accountability have grown continually worse. In the end, by following the guidance of the central government, we can focus on the proper way of financial operations of local self-governing bodies. Recent trends need to be checked and new systematic reorganization is necessary to ensure autonomy and accountability. Establishing an effective method and strategy is needed. When it comes to the issue of financial decentralization, we need to be on the lookout for issues of reckless 'politicizing' as well as reckless centralization. From the 1960s when regional financial law was established and to the present, the decentralization of regional finances has been theoretically aiming at escaping from the national financial regulations and management systems of the Ministry of Financial Planning. The establishment of general financial standards for the decentralization of an individual region's financial laws have become more and more responsible for their regional populations. However, in reality, from the planning of regional finances, decentralization and policy self-governance have headed in a centralized direction. Thus, there is a clear need for theoretical revision and systematic reform. From the vertical governance valued by the central government, a shift to horizontal governance, based on local citizens and community, needs to be established. If the governance is not prepared well, efforts for community well-being are irrational in the view of accountability. In addition, selfish leaders and bureaucrats as well as the citizens in collectivism can aggravate these efforts further. Accordingly, only after fulfilling the preconditions of democracy, we can reap the benefits of economic efficiency and accountability from pursuit for community well-being. At the root of the various criticisms and worries concerning community well-being is the issue of the loss of public consciousness and accountability of financial resources.

9.5.2 Accountability for Well-Being

Based on the debate over the transformation of policy values, the idea of accountability is fluid and can change variously depending on the environment. In the 1970s, the focus was on process and legal accountability, and in the 1980s, this focus shifted to the accountability of decentralized organizations, like managerial accountability. Afterwards, in the 1990s, consumer accountability as well as market and contract management became the focus and in the 2000s, while the idea of collective accountability was developed, the public nature of accountability became an issue.

The synthesis of product management, financial industry management and the value of information reform, is the generally agreed upon principle for the accountability of regional well-being. That is, because "regional populations, or one could say, the results and intended fruits of community are important" and reforms in local financial management are needed. Also, the special burden of local financial accountability needs to be considered. In addition, through such considerations, a needed plan for increasing the accountability can be developed.

First, the Ministry of Government Affairs and Home Affairs through various ministries and offices may manage all regional finances together. In this way, both regulation and support of regional finances are accomplished. Through the Ministry of Financial Planning's evaluation, the ministries and offices of the central government are responsible for the results of project assistance. Related to this, on the basis of vertical business operations or related indications, the duties of the regional self-governing bodies are constrained by ministry policy efforts. Second, local government own the financial accountability. In this way, local financial accountability has received much influence from the internal policy and managerial processes of the accountability structure. Traditionally, within the levels of management for financial operations, there are strategies and standards for efficiency. However, during the decades of the renovations of new public management, the accountability for the intended goals of financial operations became more deeply established. Representative financial management methods are performance budgeting based on program estimate forms. Third, governmental accountability is divided into central and local parts. This is based on common financial accountability derived from the central government's power and the regional political accountability, which is centered on the regional assembly. From a political perspective, accountability of financial operations do not agree with general financial standards. As concern to formal outcome accountability, the purposes and individual political accountability may vary. Based on local financial accountability, with an optimal division of scarce local financial resources, the realization of financial management goals themselves are possible by creating an accountability structure. The establishment of the system for well-being actually involves more issues because the accountability is surrounded and entangled in diverse political economic relations.

9.5.3 Institutional Design

Third World decentralization reforms had failed to solve the issue of accountability as it relates to the supply of services based on the residents' desire. Thus, the local democracy cannot function in an orderly fashion. From this follows many criticisms of the limited accountability of local public servants and local leaders. In local elections, under their political economic restrictions, it is easy for political leaders to seize blind benefits for the larger voting group, and to offer no effort to improve public service quality. In this way, the accountability, effectiveness and equity of decentralized public services deteriorate.

We should rebuild the decision making system of local welfare in the view of residents 'real needs and public interests in order to acquire effectiveness. First, residents' needs at the community level should be input to the local program budget properly. Effectiveness and priority are determinative for the citizens accessing political decisions for their participation. If these are low, the benefits of decentralization will not be attained. If the premise of democratization has not been attained, the local elites can easily manipulate the priority of programs. However, these reforms are difficult in local government because each preference is part of a larger public interest. Second, residents must be provided with concrete information about the improvement of living conditions. In any case, such information is not provided successfully because it is not easy for citizens to control the information thoroughly. In this context, the improved effectiveness and accountability of the program cannot be guaranteed. Thus, we should redesign the welfare budget process in terms of residents' real benefit and public interest.

9.6 Conclusions

In order to promote residents accountability to local programs, there is nothing more important than reform of the financial relations among governments. From the perspective of the central government, in order for all of the various local financial laws to agree with residents' real benefit and public interest, a comprehensive reform of all aspects of local financial law is needed. Before the revival of regional self-governance, local financial affairs were protected through central financial planning. Independent local financial operating systems of self-governing bodies were also established as a premise of local autonomy. However, at that time, vertical financial regulation of the Ministry of Home Affairs was based on a legal framework. Financial reforms were also not part of the performance budgeting. The current local financial law as focused on decentralization needs to be revised so as to accord with current residents will and public interests. When considering the needed systematic provisions, or perhaps even the founding of new provisions, the community level accountability building is the first priority. In order to reestablish the basic structure, revision of local expenditure programs is important. This is because if local programs are not performed as appropriate for latent residents' real desire and public interest, holding the related financial accountability is impossible. Also, in the big picture, the active individual subsidy operations of the national treasury can be handed over to local governments. There can be overlap in the welfare operations of the central and local governments. In such cases, the business priority of local autonomous bodies is maintained and the overlapping operations of central government must be redirected to what they are designed for. Unfortunately, the central government tends to grant financial accountability directly to regional businesses rather than to autonomous governments. The Ministry of the Treasury should adopt a more egalitarian contracting method that grants accountability to regional governments based on their results. From the perspective of financial accountability, the biggest point of contention is the mistrust with local government and local collectivism. The central government financial management system is combined with a kind of nationalism, which is concomitant strengthening of the central governments' regulations. Thus, changes are needed both in how local financial systems cultivate the autonomy of citizens and the orientation of community well-being.

First, performance evaluation indexes of the local governments should be shifted towards residents benefit and public interest. So far, most performance evaluation indexes are the check list for the process of budget expenditure and the results of output level performed by local civil servants. Second, citizen participation should be easier through exhaustive information announcements of the regional program and budget. In the dimension of social movements, the expected results in the view of residents are not guaranteed. One could say that the basis of community's democratic consciousness becomes confirmed by awakening of residents for their real benefits. Third, long term well-being plans of a diverse community level needs to be developed. The open access to statistical information as well as structural information of financial projects needs to be shared with the public. Because the degree of understanding of citizens could not be deep in the outcome accountability, participation of private experts might strengthen the validity of analysis and monitoring concerning outcomes.

Acknowledgements This work was supported by the National Research Foundation of Korea Grant funded by the Korean Government (NRF-2013S1A3A2054622).

References

Alvarez-Diaz, A., Gonzalez, L., & Radcliff, B. (2010). The politics of happiness: On the political determinants of quality of life in the American states. *The Journal of Politics, 72*(3), 894

Babula, E., & Mrzyglod, U. (2013). Economic determinants of happiness among European nations. *International Journal of Academic Research, 5*(3), 519–524.

Choi, Y. C. (2008). Relationships between national competitiveness and decentralization, Korean Association of Local Government Studies Summer Conference Proceedings.

Cox, D., Frere, M., West, S., & Wiseman, J. (2010). Developing and using local community well-being Indicators: Learning from the experience of Community Indicators Victoria. *Australian Journal of Social Issues, 45*(1), Autumn.

Easterlin, R. A. (1974). Does economic growth improve the human lot? Some empirical evidence. In P. David & M. Reder (Eds.), *Nations and households in economic growth: Essays in honour of Moses Abramovitz* (pp. 89–125). Academic Press.

Forrest, R., & Kearns, A. (2001). Social cohesion, social capital and the neighbourhood. *Urban Studies, 38*(12), 2125–2143.

Han, S., Kim, H., Lee, E.-S., & Lee, H. S. (2013). The contextual and compositional associations of social capital and subjective happiness: A multilevel analysis from Seoul, South Korea. *Journal of Happiness Studies, 14,* 1183–1200.

Helliwell, J., Huang, H., & Wang, S. (2014). Social capital and well-being in times of crisis. *Journal of Happiness Studies, 15,* 145–162.

Hewitt, J. P. (1998). *The myth of self-esteem: Finding happiness and solving problems in America.* St: Martin's Press.

Klein, C. (2013). Social capital or social cohesion: What matters for subjective well-being? *Social Indicators Research, 110,* 891–911.

Kraut, R. (1979). Two conceptions of happiness. *The Philosophical Review,* 167–197.

Lee, Y. K., & Dong K. K. (2007). A Study on the Quality of Life of Local Residents. Korean Policy Science Bulletin, *11*(4), 223–250.

Lee, T. J., Park, C. M. & Song, K. S. (2005) Analysis of quality of life of local residents, *Korean Local Government Review, 12*(4), 75–92.

Leung, A., Kier, C., Fung, T., Fung, L., & Sproule, R. (2011). Searching for happiness: The importance of social capital. *Journal of Happiness Studies, 12,* 443–462.

OECD. (2014). *How's life in your region? Measuring regional and local well-being for policy making*. Paris: OECD.

Putnam, R. D. (1993). The prosperous community: Social capital and public life. *The American Prospect, 4*(13), 1–11.

Rath, T., & Harter, J. (2010). *Well-being-the five essential elements*. New York: Gallup Press.

Soh, J. K. (1998) Definition of quality of life and its policy implications for urban policy, *Regional Community Development Review, 23*(1), 65–84.

White, S. (2008). But what is Well-being? In *A framework for analysis in social and development policy and practice* (pp. 3–7). University of Bradford.

Wiseman, J., & Brasher, K. (2008). Community well-being in an unwell World: Trends, challenges, and possibilities. *Journal of Public Health Policy, 29*(3), 353–366.

Youngkyun Oh is Professor in the Department of Public Administration at Suwon University. He is charged with Dean of Human & Social Science and Dean of Public Administration Graduate School. Currently, he serves on the editorial board of Springer's Community Quality-of-Life and Well-Being book series. His research interests include Korea Public Administration, Regional Public Management and research and development policy.

Chapter 10
Arts and Community Well-Being

HeeKyung Sung

Abstract This chapter reviews a broad array of community well-being literature and then specifies the dimensions of community well-being (i.e., individual, social, and economic well-being). Also, the notion of arts and cultural impacts within community well-being dimensions is discussed from several different perspectives. Specifically, this chapter provides an overview of the general concept of community well-being. A number of arts and cultural components that influence community well-being are then discussed. Lastly, based on the literature, this chapter proposes a conceptual model of arts and community well-being which can be used to examine the relationship between arts and cultural assets and community well-being outcomes.

Keywords Arts · Community well-being · Culture · Cultural assets · Social well-being

10.1 Introduction

Arts and culture function as indispensable parts of humans' lives. Numerous studies have examined the impact and value of arts and culture, from individual quality of life to overall community health. However, research has been less focused on identifying the influence of crucial dimensions of arts and culture on overall community well-being and contributing to understanding the intertwining connection between these elements and community well-being. This chapter is to explore the dimensions of arts and cultural resources and community well-being, and in turn, to develop a conceptual framework in order to present the relationship between them in a community. To understand the relationship between arts and community well-being, a general concept of community well-being is presented first. When we envision a concept of community well-being, people may agree that community well-being is reflected by a wide range of economic, social, environmental, cultural, human, and political

H. Sung (✉)
Department of Recreation and Tourism Management, California State University, Northridge, CA 91330, USA
e-mail: heekyung.sung@csun.edu

© Springer Nature Switzerland AG 2019

Y. Kee et al. (eds.), *Perspectives on Community Well-Being*, Community Quality-of-Life and Well-Being, https://doi.org/10.1007/978-3-030-15115-7_10

forces. Also, the well-being of a community is reflected in aspects of personal life and residents' satisfaction. Residents, especially at the local level, play an essential role in determining the economic, social and cultural prosperity (Insch & Florek, 2008) and collective outcomes of residents regarding various economic, social, and physical statuses that can be considered evidence of community well-being.

To put it another way, community well-being can encompass residents' quality of life and related community conditions. From the community perspective, while there is no one universal definition, the premise of the well-being of a community is "enhancing, creating or recreating healthy and viable communities" (Christakopoulou, Dawson, & Gari, 2001, p. 321). Much literature defines community well-being within similar boundaries. For example, the Local Government Community Services Association of Australia (lGCSAA) defines community well-being as "qualities for developing healthy and sustainable communities" (Derrett, 2003, p. 53). Also, Wiseman and Brasher (2008) describe community well-being as "the combination of social, economic, environmental, cultural, and political conditions identified by individuals and their communities as essential for them to flourish and fulfill their potential" (p. 358).

10.2 Exploring Community Well-Being

Some researchers consider community well-being as subjective resident satisfaction regarding a local place. Whorton and Moore (1984) argued that collective and subjective information serve as reasonable indicators for community satisfaction, and then discussed six core community satisfaction concepts included concern for crime, concern for the availability of jobs, concern for access to adequate health care, concern for available housing, satisfaction with public education, and satisfaction with community (p. 299). Forjaz et al. (2011) suggested that satisfaction with the local place of residence entails the social and physical environment, community services and facilities, and attachment to community. They claimed that community well-being is an important indicator to gauge the impact of local community on peoples' health and general well-being and develop a community well-being index that included eleven items.

On the other hand, Wills (2001) posited that the ultimate goal of community well-being is to make a community successful in balancing between environmental sustainability, economic prosperity, and outcomes such as livability, equity, vitality, sustainability, and prosperity. Furthermore, she held that in order for a community to achieve the state of wellness, good governance is essential. Following this, Cuthill (2004) claimed, "community well-being is the ultimate goal of all democratic governance including that delivered by local government" (p. 9). He emphasized that building human and social capital achieved by citizen participation is critical as a basis for community well-being. In a similar manner, a research study conducted by Finlay, Hardy, Morris, and Nagy (2010) posited that social factors (e.g., education, employment and working conditions, health care services, housing, social safety, communications, and special factors based on community context) are essential for understanding community wellness. According to their research, these factors are related to community health outcomes, especially in a distressed community, and improvements of these factors influence the rebuilding of a community which is embodied in community well-being.

Another approach focusing on social factors can be found in the study of Maybery, Pope, Hodgins, Hitchenor, and Shepherd (2009). Specifically, they approach community well-being as community resilience of residents coping with their stressful circumstances. In this study, key ecological factors that influence resilient communities are social assets, service assets that support community action and behavior, neighborhood and economic resources, and community risk factors such as levels of crime. As a result of a survey of small inland rural communities in Australia, it demonstrates that social assets are the most valued in the community as a way to build community well-being. Again, it supports the claim that social connectedness and social ties are critical determinants for community resilience and well-being.

Furthermore, the burgeoning literature in Australia seeks to provide an integrated understanding of local community well-being (Cox, Frere, West, & Wiseman, 2010; Davern, West, Bodenham, & Wiseman, 2011; Miles, Greer, Kraatz, & Kinnear, 2008; Wills, 2001; Wiseman & Brasher, 2008; Wiseman et al. 2006). Their focus goes beyond individual and collective well-being and moves on to the circumstances and outcomes of the broader community. Wills (2001) proposed three community domains (i.e., social, economic, and environmental domains) linked to seven community well-being outcomes, including livability, equity, conviviality, vitality, adequate prosperity, sustainability, and viability.

Miles et al. (2008) developed a model to measure community well-being. The model is referred to as the six-by-six community well-being model. It is comprised of six dimensions featuring 36 indicators, with each dimension consisting of six indicators to cover economic, social, and environmental well-being in a community. The six dimensions include: (1) wealth and affordability, (2) safety and public health, (3) personal health and fitness, (4) diversity and learning, (5) community and governance, and (6) environment and infrastructure. Based on these six dimensions, they suggested that community well-being indicators could reflect a community's health and its basic quality of life and be used as a tool for better understanding of status quo of the community in relation to other communities.

Similarly, Wiseman and Brasher (2008), Cox et al. (2010), and Davern et al, (2011), presented the Community Indicators Victoria (CIV) commissioned by the Victorian Health Promotion Foundation (VicHealth) as a tool for measuring well-being of a local community. The CIV provides a broad picture of progress and well-being of community, combining not only subjective measures but also objective ones in five overarching domains:

- Health, safe and inclusive communities
- Dynamic, resilient economies
- Sustainable built and natural environment

- Culturally rich and vibrant communities
- Democratic and engaged communities

More interestingly, CIV regarded arts and cultural activities, sporting and recreational activities, and cultural diversity as important components for community well-being. These indicators are included in the domain titled "culturally rich and vibrant communities."

There are several other instruments that are broadly linked to community well-being, although these are established to measure the state of cities and communities from the perspective of well-being and sustainability. The City Monitor was initiated by the Department of Urban Policy of the central Flemish administrative organization in Belgium (Van Asseche, Block, & Reynaert, 2010). They agitated that indicators simplify the representation of societal problems, and in this manner, they proposed a sustainability framework (The City Monitor) to map livable signs of Flemish cities. The City Monitor is based on the concept of sustainability, focusing on economic, social, physical-ecological, and institutional principles; these sustainability principles interrelate eight activity domains that can take place in the city such as living, education, working, safety, social welfare, culture, environment, and mobility. As community indicators, the implementation of the City Monitor helped analyze the quality of life in Flemish communities (Van Asseche et al. 2010).

On the other hand, Michalos et al. (2011) offer a different take on the well-being concept by suggesting a Canadian Index of Wellbeing (CIW). Even though their primary goal was to measure a composite index of well-being, they posited that most of the phenomena relevant to well-being at the present time could be conceptualized in eight domains. As shown in Fig. 10.1, each domain of the CIW system is symbolized in three resources (i.e., personal, public, and ecosystem resources). For example, the personal resources for well-being includes resources in order to achieve personal well-being; that is, healthy populations, time use, and education. The second concentric circle presents public resources that encompass living standards, demographic engagement, community vitality, and leisure and culture. As an ecosystem resource, the environment affects all of the domains. The authors noted that the CIW system illustrates the general shape of domains and interaction among all the circles occurs to sustain well-being.

Lastly, the County Health Ranking and Roadmaps (CHRR) was developed as a collaborative work between the Robert Wood Johnson Foundation and the University of Wisconsin Population Health Institute to measure community vital health factors in nearly every county in the United States (County health ranking and roadmaps (CHRR), n. d.). It provides a reliable, sustainable source of local data to communities to help them identify opportunities to improve their community health. The health factors emphasized were divided into health behaviors and clinical care (e.g., diet and exercise, smoking, and access to physicians), social and economic factors (e.g., education, crime rate, and employment), and physical environment (e.g., air and water quality, housing, and transit); these factor influence a multi-dimensional concept of quality of life that includes domains related to physical, mental, emotional, and social functioning.

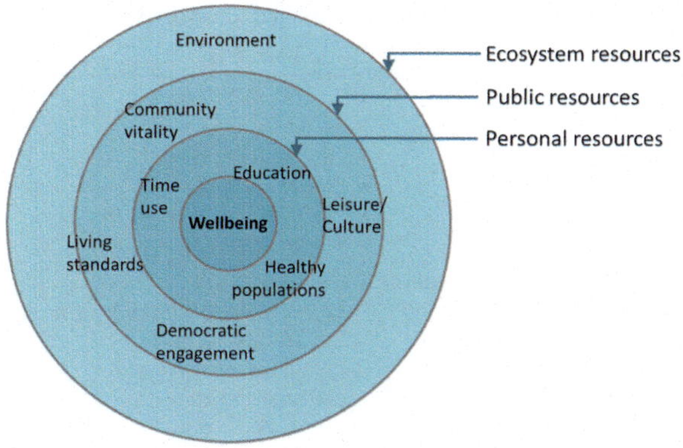

Fig. 10.1 The Mandala of wellbeing adapted from Michalos et al. (2011, p. 7)

Given the above rationale, it is recognized that the concept of community well-being is grounded in not only the residents' perceptions and satisfaction to the community but also on community conditions, qualities, and assets. The aforementioned studies focusing on identifying components that were comprehensive and consistent across the communities also offered intriguing insights into how community indicators are developed and used to gauge current community well-being. Sung and Phillips (2018) posit that community indicators are small pieces of information which combines with other pieces of information so as to convey a picture of the situation in a community. In particular, community well-being indicators focus on not only the engagement of local residents but also community strengthening. Ultimately, indicators provides comprehensive and useful information that informs community priorities and the status of a community (Phillips, 2003). In other words, community well-being indicators can help us measure the levels of community well-being, identify goals and needs, track progress towards goals, and strengthen community competencies (Sung & Phillips, 2018). Thus, the following section shows how a range of aspects affecting the state of a local community are categorized under the community well-being studies, focusing more on various community well-being dimensions and subsequent measurements.

10.3 Measuring Community Well-Being

As a framework for community assessment, community well-being should be reflected by a range of aspects affecting the state of a local community. A number of studies suggested a range of community well-being indicators with multidimensional aspects of well-being as a viable proxy for community (the majority have been discussed in the previous section). These are summarized below in Table 10.1.

As in the community well-being literature, empirical investigations of community well-being have examined the effects of several objective and subjective items.

Table 10.1 Summary of studies related to community well-being (CWB) measurement

Studies	Domain of CWB	Measurement indicators
Whorton and Moore (1984)	• Concern for crime • Availability of jobs • Concern for health care • Concern for housing • Satisfaction with public education • Satisfaction with community	*Focus on subjective measurement* • Total 24 items to present six core factors, with each factor comprising four items
Christakopoulou et al. (2001)	• Place to live (a) Satisfaction with built environment (b) Service and facilities (c) Environmental quality (d) Personal safety • Social community (a) Community spirit (b) Informal interaction • Economic community (a) Income sufficiency • Political community (a) Decision making process • Personal space (a) Place attachment • Part of the city	*Focus on subjective and objective measurement* • Total 45 items to present nine sub-domains
Wills (2001)	• Social/physical well-being • Economic well-being • Environmental well-being	• Economic development • Environmental sustainability • Public/environmental health • Community safety • Housing • Physical, emotional social and spiritual development • Social determinants of health
Cuthill (2004)	• Social capital • Human capital • Physical capital • Financial capital • Natural capital	• The cohesiveness of people and societies • The status of individuals • Local infrastructure including education, housing, and health services • Stocks of money, savings, and pensions • Nature's goods and services
Cox et al. (2010), Davern et al. (2011), and Wiseman et al. (2006)	Community Indicator Victoria • Healthy, safe, and inclusive communities • Dynamic, resilient and fair economies • Sustainable built and natural environments • Culturally rich and vibrant communities • Democratic and active citizenship	*Focus on subjective and objective measurement* • Multi-item scales in terms of 23 sub-domains and 72 indicators

(continued)

Table 10.1 (continued)

Studies	Domain of CWB	Measurement indicators
Miles et al. (2008)	• Wealth and Affordability • Safety and Public Heath • Personal health and Fitness • Diversity and Learning • Community and Governance • Environment and Infrastructure	*Focus on subjective and objective measurement* • Total 36 items to present six core factors, with each factor comprising six items
Maybery et al. (2009)	• Social assets • Service agency assets • Neighborhood and economic resources • Community risks	*Focus on subjective measurement* • Total 20 items 17 asset typed items and 3 items of common risk types of community
Finlay et al. (2010)	Emphasis on northern First Nations in Canada • Social determinants of health • Factors with respect to the northern context, including First Nations cultural perspectives	*Focus on subjective measurement* • 13 sub-domains of social determinants of health (e.g., education, employment, food security, health care services, social safety, etc.) • 8 factors regarding First Nations context (e.g., colonization, territory, poverty, cultural continuity, etc.)
Van Asseche et al. 2010	The City Monitor (1) Eight activity domains Living • Learning and education • Care and welfare • Culture and leisure • Working and enterprise • Safety and protection • Transportation and mobility • Nature and environment (2) Four sustainable principles • Economic principles • Social principles • Physical-ecological principles • Institutional principles	• 200 indicators from statistics, registrations, surveys, and other data sources
Sirgy et al. (2010)	• Social well-being • Leisure well-being • Health well-being • Safety well-being • Family and home well-being • Political well-being • Spiritual well-being • Neighborhood well-being • Environmental well-being • Transportation well-being • Education well-being • Work well-being • Financial well-being • Consumer well-being	*Focus on subjective measurement* • 87 multi-items based on 14 domains

(continued)

Table 10.1 (continued)

Studies	Domain of CWB	Measurement indicators
White (2010)	• The material • The social • The human	*Focus on subjective and objective measurement* • Practical welfare and standards of living • Social relations and public goods • Capabilities, values and attitudes
Michalos et al. (2011)	Canadian Index of Wellbeing (1) Personal resources • Healthy populations • Time use • Education (2) Public resources • Living standards • Community vitality • Democratic engagement • Leisure and culture (3) Ecosystem resources • Environment	• Total 64 items to present eight core factors, with each factor comprising eight items
Forjaz et al. (2011)	• Community services • Community attachment • Physical and social environment	*Focus on subjective measurement* • Support to families • Social services • Leisure • Health services • Security • Belonging • Trust in people • Social conditions • Economic situation • Environment
County Health Rankings and Roadmaps (n.d.)	• Health outcomes • Health behaviors • Clinical care • Social and economic factors • Physical environment	• Total 36 items under the 16 sub-domains of determinants of community health (e.g., education, employment, diet and exercise, safety, social support, etc.)

Source Adapted and modified from Sung, Table 17 (2016, p. 94) and from Sung and Phillips (2018)

Community well-being can be driven by residents' subjective quality of life in that if people are satisfied with their living conditions in a community, the community will be more likely to reach a status of well-being. On the other hand, if the community endeavors to develop infrastructure and community systems, this can also influence the quality of life of residents, and in turn, impact community well-being. Overall, the community well-being assessment was built on a mix of indicators such as personal physical and mental health, education, poverty, unemployment, and crime. In other words, potential data assessing community well-being can be derived from not only peoples' perceived evaluation of their life circumstances, but also from objective indices which are publicly collected in the communities. Also, while there is some dispute in the literature regarding the definition and operationalization of community well-being, as well as the construction of its system, domains and a variety of characteristics can be classified into more general dimensions. Taken the studies illustrated in the Table 10.1 as a whole, important components for community well-being can be parsed in physical (human), economic, social, and environmental contexts. The following offers four distinct ways of characterizing community well-being:

- *Physical (individual) community well-being* refers to the well-being aspects of personal health and nutrition associated with the state of physical and mental health. With respect to characteristics, indicators could be physical activity, smoking and drug use, obesity, and mental and physical health of residents.
- *Social community well-being* refers to well-being outcomes derived from relation-dynamics in a community. It includes social networks, inclusion, safety, and community formation indicators such as voting rate, crime rate, education attainment, and volunteering rate.
- *Economic community well-being* encompasses the economic state of the community. Economic well-being is reflected in income levels, housing quality, employment, and investment and spending patterns.
- *Environmental community well-being* embraces nature-related dimensions of community infrastructures. Furthermore, it also covers overall living environments associated with physical, social, and economic well-being components in a community.

It is difficult to find and measure all the constituents and determinants that impact community well-being system. Also, the function of each community well-being dimension based on the above literature can overlap and interact with each other. In many discussions of community well-being, there is not enough attention paid to the role of arts and cultural assets, while much literature from arts and cultural industry fields claims arts impact on residents' and community quality of life. To see a broad, as well as detailed image of the relationship between community well-being and arts and cultural capacity, the next section focuses more on synthesizing arts and cultural values and impacts within community well-being context. While there are many other variables that influence community well-being, this chapter explores it in the context of a focus on art-community well-being relationships.

10.3.1 Arts and Culture Connections to Community Well-Being

Community well-being is grounded in community conditions, qualities, and assets that are derived from community characteristics. Arts and culture are embodied in, or at least related to, human and community life. It seems that arts and cultural assets and residents' consumptions of these are linked to community well-being, despite the lack of attention on the impacts of arts and culture in community well-being studies. A few studies related to community indicators emphasized the values of arts and culture in community well-being (Besleme, Maser, & Silverstein, 1999; Cox et al., 2010; Davern et al., 2011). Besleme et al. (1999) and introduced two local community indicators projects from Jacksonville, Florida and Truckee Meadows region in Nevada. Jacksonville indicators discuss culture and recreation as one of the ten elements of quality of life in Jacksonville, while Truckee Meadows indicators more specifically point out arts as one of the ten elements of community quality of life. Another approach can be found in Community Indicators Victoria (CIV). It evaluated cultural viability-arts and cultural activities, sporting and recreational activities, and cultural diversity-as important components for community well-being (Cox et al., 2010; Davern et al., 2011). Although they did not quote community well-being directly, it was found that much research has examined the relationship between arts and various well-being components of a community such as residents' health, social networks, civic engagement, and economic prosperity (Catterall, 2012; Daykin et al., 2013; Grodach, 2011; Hayter & Pierce, 2009; Michalos & Kahlke, 2010; Rogers & Anastasiadou, 2011). Table 10.2 summarizes a wide range of arts and cultural benefits related to community well-being (CWB).

In this sense, promoting artistic and cultural environments synthetically influence overall community well-being. Furthermore, as a result of prior factor analysis conducted based on 17 local arts indicators with 518 counties in U.S, the ABCN (Arts Business, Consumption, and Nonprofit) framework was indicated that arts business, arts consumption, and arts nonprofit could be essential components to measure the vitality of arts and culture in a community (Sung, 2016). Given that, accordance with the ABCN and community well-being components, Fig. 10.2 illustrates how arts and cultural resources are synthesized in the context of community well-being.

This diagram demonstrates how diverse factors of arts and culture are related to and have potential to make contributions toward community well-being. A few details about the arts and cultural indicators of each domain include:

Table 10.2 Summary of arts and cultural impact related to community well-being

Physical (individual) well-being	Social well-being	Economic well-being
• Achieve hedonic pleasure or aesthetic appreciation • Build artistic skills • Promote physical and psychological health • Cultivate self-expression • Improve self-confidence and self esteem • Increase creativity	• Reduce youth delinquency • Build social relationships and networks • Enhance civic engagement • Develop community cohesion • Support social inclusion • Improve community cooperation • Understand local identity and culture • Encourage community empowerment	• Generate employment • Yield arts products • Promote arts consumption • Forster artists and arts industries • Promote a city's image • Foster local businesses and services • Support nonprofit organizations and facilities

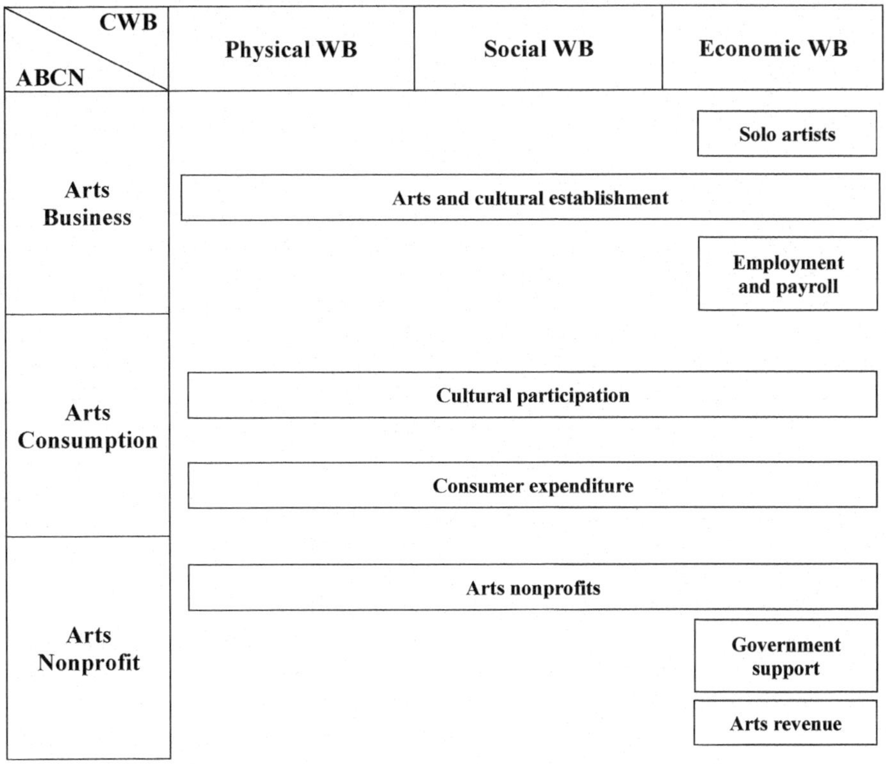

Fig. 10.2 A diagram of the evidence of arts and cultural contribution to CWB

- *Arts Business* refers to the level of arts businesses related to a direct economic impact on arts and cultures in a community. With respect to characteristics, indicators could be arts/cultural share of all payroll; arts/cultural share of all employees; creative industry share of all employees; arts/cultural establishments; creative industry businesses; and solo artists.
- *Arts Consumption* refers to the consumption of arts and cultural facilities and resources in a community. It includes photographic equipment expenditures; entertainment admission fees; recorded media expenditures; online music purchase; attending live performance; and musical instruments expenditures. It helps estimate the number of people engaged in and how much money they spend on art-related activities. Furthermore, it provides insight into the scope of the arts and cultural market through participation and expenditures by the local population.
- *Arts Nonprofit* encompasses the overall scope of the nonprofit arts sectors in a community. With respect to characteristics, indicators could be collections-based nonprofits; humanities/heritage nonprofits; state arts agency grants; total nonprofit arts revenue; and performing/events nonprofits. It helps provide insight into the prosperity of the arts and cultural market in a community.

Fig. 10.3 Arts and community well-being excerpted and modified from "how art works" illustrated by Iyengar et al. (2012, p. 17)

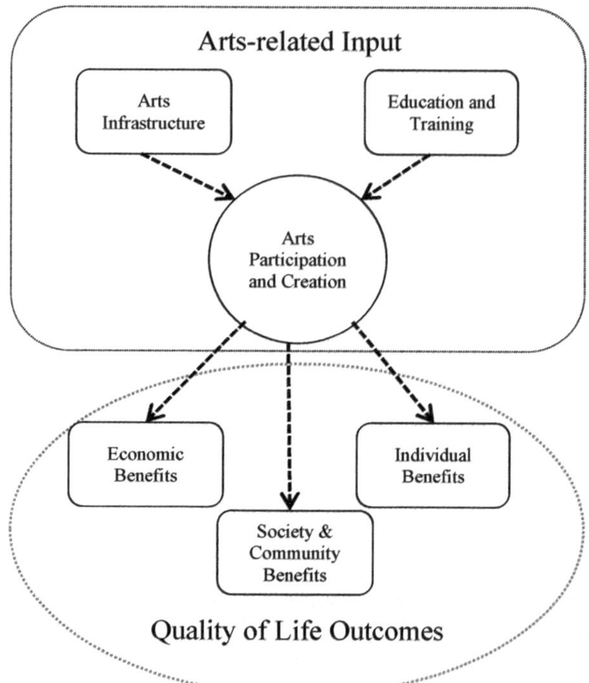

In addition, the "how art works" system map constructed by Iyengar et al. (2012) shows a clear vision with respect to arts-related inputs and direct and indirect community outcomes. In particular, focusing on art inputs and quality of life outcomes in this system (see Fig. 10.3), arts infrastructure and arts-related education and training invigorate arts creation and participation, and in turn, these arts-related inputs influence individuals, society, and communities, and direct and indirect economic outputs. Therefore, in consideration of aforementioned discussions, it could be proposed that interactions between arts and each well-being dimension have some influence on overall community well-being environment.

However, to operationalize the conceptual framework presented in the following, there are some gaps in previous empirical studies. For example, arts infrastructure, and arts education and training influence primarily arts participation rather than other community outcomes. Although their claim that arts infrastructure and education impact arts participation and creation is obvious, others argue that arts infrastructure such as arts organizations and arts venue also can be used as a tool for community economic development (Grodach, 2010, 2011; Hayter & Pierce, 2009; Lavanga, 2006; Markusen & Gadwa, 2010).

Also, arts education and training influence not only the likelihood of arts participation and creation, but also, as an independent factor, are related to the individual and social benefits. Ruppert (2006) and others (Catterall, 2012; Respress & Lutfi, 2006; Walker, 1995) indicate that arts learning is of benefit to students, supporting their academic success and reducing youth delinquency. Furthermore, Bailey, Miles, and Stark (2004) examine how art works and programs in areas of social deprivation support community revitalization, gathering the collective ability to relieve social problems and increase capacity. Lastly, according to Sung (2016), arts business, arts consumption, and arts nonprofit domains encompass the essential attributes of arts and culture in the context of community environment. Therefore, on the basis of all things considered, a model for investigating the relationship between the arts and community well-being can be proposed.

10.3.2 Arts and Community Well-Being Model

The purpose of this chapter is to explore the relationship between key domains of arts and culture and community outcomes in the context of community well-being. The conceptual model for this study was initiated by drawing a simple relationship (see Fig. 10.4). Determination and construction of key variables with consistent and interpretable data are imperative to understand comprehensive phenomena regarding arts and community. Previous community well-being literature and Local Arts Index (LAI) reports helped construct a concrete model to gauge arts' value and impact on the lives of individuals and communities.

As a next step, to measure arts and cultural resources, categorizing these into key factors was important. Drawing on the Local Arts Index, Sung (2016) identified three underlying dimensions of arts and culture: arts business (e.g., artists, arts and cultural establishment, employee, and payroll), arts consumption (e.g., arts participation and consumption), and arts nonprofit (e.g., nonprofit arts revenues and government support). Given that, Fig. 10.5 suggests that the core dimensions with supporting indicators were suggested in the left box. Furthermore, outcomes of community well-being are dependent variables in this conceptual model. From the previous literature, community well-being is accounted by the multicultural character of communities (see Table 10.1). However, with consideration for the notable well-being domains related to arts and culture, this study covers individual, social, and economic well-being variables.

In effect, this model will investigate a more complicated relationship between arts and cultural resources and outcomes of community well-being. Based upon an understanding of the impact of arts and culture on community, this study argues that each arts and cultural dimension influences outcomes of community

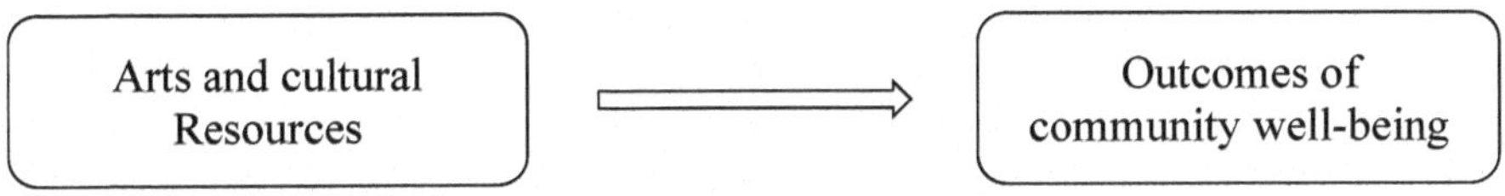

Fig. 10.4 The relationship between arts and community

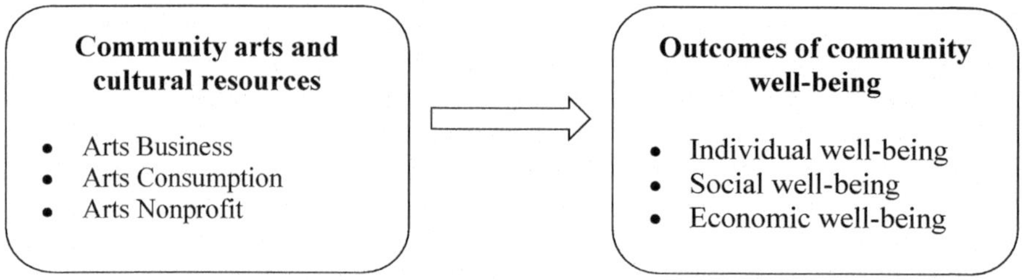

Fig. 10.5 The model of arts and community well-being

well-being. Furthermore, these might selectively support specific dimensions of community well-being. For example, arts business might be related to economic community well-being outcome rather than individual well-being. On the other hand, arts consumption might broadly influence all three dimensions of community well-being. Given that, the present research considers whether or not arts and cultural resources of local communities positively affect community human, social, economic outcomes, and, by extension, collective well-being which combines above three well-being components at the county level, examining my broadest research question "if a community has more abundant arts and cultural resources and activities, does it have better community well-being?" Therefore, the expanded model and propositions are as follows (see Fig. 10.6):

Proposition 1: *With an abundant presence of arts and cultural assets within a community, community individual well-being will be positively enhanced.*

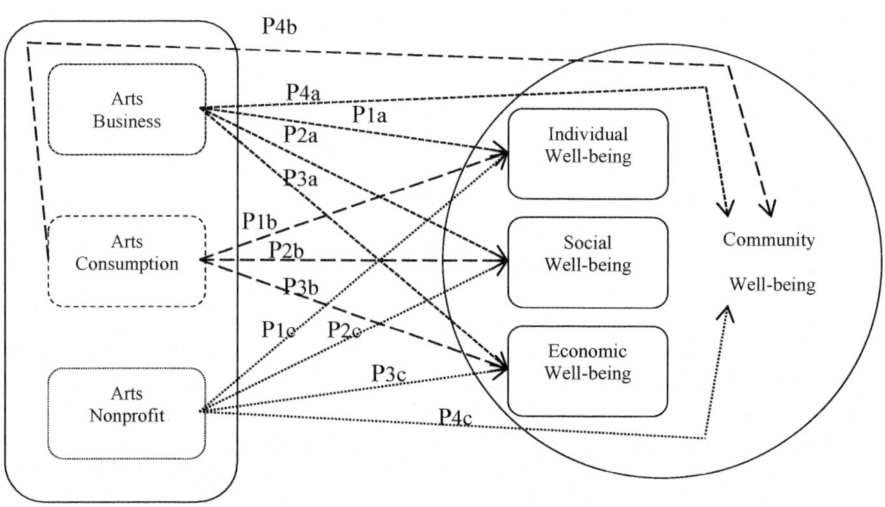

Fig. 10.6 An expanded model of arts and community well-being

Proposition 1a: With an abundant presence of arts and cultural business factors within a community, community individual well-being will be positively enhanced.
Proposition 1b: Peoples' arts and cultural consumptions and experiences have a positive impact on community individual well-being outcomes.
Proposition 1c: With an abundant presence of arts and cultural nonprofit factors within a community, community individual well-being will be positively enhanced.

Proposition 2: *With an abundant presence of arts and cultural assets within a community, community social well-being will be positively enhanced.*

Proposition 2a: With an abundant presence of arts and cultural business factors within a community, community social well-being will be positively enhanced.
Proposition 2b: Peoples' arts and cultural consumptions and experiences have a positive impact on community social well-being outcomes.
Proposition 2c: With an abundant presence of arts and cultural nonprofit factors within a community, community social well-being will be positively enhanced.

Proposition 3: *With an abundant presence of arts and cultural assets within a community, community economic well-being will be positively enhanced.*

Proposition 3a: With an abundant presence of arts and cultural business factors within a community, community economic well-being will be positively enhanced.
Proposition 3b: Peoples' arts and cultural consumptions and experiences have a positive impact on community economic well-being outcomes.
Proposition 3c: With an abundant presence of arts and cultural nonprofit factors within a community, community economic well-being will be positively enhanced.

Proposition 4: *With an abundant presence of arts and cultural assets within a community, overall community well-being will be positively enhanced.*

Proposition 4a: With an abundant presence of arts and cultural business factors within a community, overall community well-being will be positively enhanced.
Proposition 4b: Peoples' arts and cultural consumptions and experiences have a positive impact on overall community well-being outcomes.
Proposition 4c: With an abundant presence of arts and cultural nonprofit factors within a community, overall community well-being will be positively enhanced.

10.4 Summary

This chapter reviewed a broad array of community well-being literature and the dimensions of community well-being (i.e., individual, social, and economic well-being) and their measurement system was discussed. Also, this chapter proposed a conceptualization of the arts and community well-being model. It included a number of propositions that focus on the impact of the arts and cultural resource dimensions in a community on the individual, social, and economic outcomes within a county level. Specifically, in line with the result of the factor analysis drawn from prior studies

(Local arts index (LAX), n.d.; Sung, 2016), it is postulated that arts and cultural business, consumption, and nonprofit factors influence local individual, social, and economic outcomes, which reflect different dimensions of community well-being. We present the propositions in this chapter to encourage further research and thinking on the ideas around connections between arts and community well-being. While much more work is needed on development of measurements and constructs for gauging community well-being, this chapter serves to foster additional insights in the context of the arts.

References

Bailey, C., Miles, S., & Stark, P. (2004). Culture-led urban regeneration and the revitalisation of identities in Newcastle, Gateshead and the North East of England. *International Journal of Cultural Policy, 10*(1), 47–65.

Besleme, K., Maser, E., & Silverstein, J. (1999). *A community indicators case study: Addressing the quality of life in two communities*. San Francisco, CA: Redefining Progress.

Catterall, J. S. (2012). *The arts and achievement in at-risk youth: Findings from four longitudinal studies Research Report# 55*. Washington, DC: National Endowment for the Arts.

Christakopoulou, S., Dawson, J., & Gari, A. (2001). The community well-being questionnaire: Theoretical context and initial assessment of its reliability and validity. *Social Indicators Research, 56,* 321–351.

County Health Rankings and Roadmaps. (n.d.). *County health rankings and roadmaps*. Retrieved from http://www.countyhealthrankings.org/about-project.

Cox, D., Frere, M., West, S., & Wiseman, J. (2010). Developing and using local community well-being indicators: Learning from the experience of community indicators Victoria. *Australian Journal of Social Issues, 45*(1), 71–88.

Cuthill, M. (2004). Community well-being: The ultimate goal of democratic governance. *Queensland Planner, 44*(2), 8–11.

Davern, M. T., West, S., Bodenham, S., & Wiseman, J. (2011). Community indicators in action: Using indicators as a tool for planning and evaluating the health and wellbeing of a community. In M. J. Sirgy, R. Phillips, & D. Rahtz (Eds.), *Community quality-of -life indicators; Best cases V* (pp. 319–338). New York: Springer Science + Business Media.

Daykin, N., Viggiani, N. D., Pilkington, P., & Moriatry, Y. (2013). Music making for health, well-being and behavior change in youth justice settings: A systematic review. *Health Promotion International, 28*(2), 197–210.

Derrett, R. (2003). Festivals and regional destinations: How festivals demonstrate a sense of community and place. *Rural Society, 13*(1), 35–53.

Finlay, J., Hardy, M., Morris, D., & Nagy, A. (2010). Mamow Ki-ken-da-ma-win: A partnership approach to Child, Youth, Family and Community wellbeing. *International Journal of Mental Health Addiction, 8,* 245–257.

Forjaz, M. J., Prieto-Flores, M. E., Ayala, A., Rodriguez-Blazquez, C., Fernandez-Mayoralas, G., Rojo-perez, F., et al. (2011). Measurement properties of the community wellbeing index in older adults. *Quality Life Research, 20,* 733–743.

Grodach, C. (2010). Art spaces, public space, and the link to community development. *Community Development Journal, 45*(4), 474–493.

Grodach, C. (2011). Art spaces in community and economic development: Connections to neighborhoods, artists, and the cultural economy. *Journal of Planning Education and Research, 31*(1), 74–85.

Hayter, C., & Pierce, S. C. (2009). *Arts & the economy: Using arts and culture to stimulate state economic development.* Washington, DC: NGA Center for Best Practices.

Insch, A., & Florek, M. (2008). A great place to live, work and play: Conceptualising place satisfaction in the case of a city's residents. *Journal of Place Management and Development, 1*(2), 138–149.

Iyengar, S., Grantham, E., Heeman, R., Ivanchenko, R., Nichols, B., Shingler, T., et al. (2012). *How art works: The National Endowment for the Arts' five-year research agenda, with a system map and measurement model.* Washington, DC: National Endowment for the Arts.

Lavanga, M. (2006). The contribution of cultural and creative industries to a more sustainable urban development: The case studies of Rotterdam and Tampere. Paper for the ACEI: *Association of cultural Economics International Conference*, Vienna, Austria, 6–9 July 2006.

Local arts index (n.d.). *Local arts index—where I live*. Retrieved from http://www.artsindexusa.org/where-i-live.

Markusen, A., & Gadwa, A. (2010). *Creative placemaking*. Washington, DC: National Endowment for the Arts.

Maybery, D., Pope, R., Hodgins, G., Hitchenor, Y., & Shepherd, A. (2009). Resilience and well-being of small inland communities: community assets as key determinants. *Rural Society, 19*(4), 326–339.

Michalos, A. C., & Kahlke, P. M. (2010). Arts and the perceived quality of life in British Columbia. *Social Indicators Research, 96,* 1–39.

Michalos, A.C., Smale, B., Labonté, R., Muharjarine, N., Scott, K., Moore, K., …, Hyman, I. (2011). *The Canadian Index of Wellbeing.* Technical Report 1.0. Waterloo, ON: Canadian Index of Wellbeing and University of Waterloo.

Miles, R. L., Greer, L., Kraatz, D., & Kinnear, S. (2008). Measuring community wellbeing: A central Queensland case study. *Australasian Journal of Regional Studies, 14*(1), 73–93.

Phillips, R. (2003). *Community indicators.* Planning Advisory Service Report 517. Chicago, IL: American Planning Association.

Respress, T., & Lutfi, G. (2006). Whole brain learning: The fine arts with students at risk. *Reclaiming Children and Youth, 15*(1), 24–31.

Rogers, P., & Anastasiadou, C. (2011). Community involvement in festivals: Exploring ways of increasing local participation. *Event Management, 15*(4), 387–399.

Ruppert, S. S. (2006). *Critical evidence: How the arts benefit student achievement.* Washington, DC: National Assembly of State Arts Agencies.

Sirgy, M. J., Widgery, R. N., Lee, D., & Yu, G. B. (2010). Developing a measure of community well-being based on perceptions of impact in various life domains. *Social Indicators Research, 96*(2), 295–311.

Sung, H. (2016). *The influence and role of arts on community well-being* (Doctoral dissertation, Arizona State University). Retrieved from https://repository.asu.edu//attachments/170292/content/Sung_asu_0010E_15684.pdf.

Sung, H., & Phillips, R. G. (2018). Indicators and community well-being: Exploring a relational framework. *International Journal of Community Well-Being, 1*(1). https://doi.org/10.1007/s42413-018-0006-0.

Van Assche, J., Block, T., & Reynaert, H. (2010). Can community indicators live up to their expectations? The case of the Flemish city monitor for livable and sustainable urban development. *Applied Research in Quality of Life, 5*(4), 341–352.

Walker, D. M. (1995). *Connecting right and left brain: Increasing academic performance of African American students through the arts.* ED 390 857.

White, S. C. (2010). Analyzing wellbeing: A framework for developing practice. *Development in Practice, 20*(2), 158–172.

Whorton, J. W., & Moore, A. B. (1984). Summative scales for measuring community satisfaction. *Social Indicators Research, 15*(3), 297–307.

Wills, J. (2001). Measuring community wellbeing: A framework for the development of community indicators. In: *Local Government Community Services Association of Australia (LGCSAA) 8th Biennial National Conference*, Perth, Australia.
Wiseman, J., & Brasher, K. (2008). Community wellbeing in an unwell world: Trends, challenges, and possibilities. *Journal of Public Health Policy, 29,* 353–366.
Wiseman, J., Heine, W., Langworthy, A., McLean, N., Pyke, J., Raysmith, H., et al. (2006). *Measuring wellbeing: Engaging communities.* Victoria, Australia: VicHealth.

HeeKyung Sung is an assistant professor in the Department of Recreation and Tourism Management at California State University, Northridge. She earned her Ph.D. from Arizona State University. Her research focuses on the impacts and value of arts and cultural events on local community and their relationships with community development and quality of life, and consumer behavior in the context of community well-being. Her published research includes studies of the community indicators, community well-being and development, consumer experiential values on local events, local art agencies in cultural tourism management. From 2006 to 2009, Sung worked as event planner at the Seongnam Performing Arts Center in Korea. Additionally, she currently has involved in the research of the experiential marketing and customer satisfaction and well-being in tourism, meeting and event industry.

Chapter 11
Spirituality: The Missing Link of Sustainability and Happiness as a Framework for Holistic Development

Erica Berejnoi, Rohana Ulluwishewa, Scott Cloutier, Leah Gibbons, Susana Puga and Anura Uthumange

Abstract There is a growing consensus that sustainability and happiness are interrelated—while happiness promotes sustainable behaviours, sustainable behaviours enhance happiness. However, there are other factors linking sustainability and happiness. In this chapter, we identify the missing link as spirituality. Our exploration differentiates spirituality from religion and presents it in rational and scientific terms and points out how individuals become intrinsically happier and behave in sustainable ways as they grow spiritually. Spirituality can be the source of both happiness and sustainability and, ultimately, enhanced community well-being. Drawing on this understanding, we then develop a theoretical framework for sustainable personal and community development that is holistic and can help foster understanding of the role of spirituality in happiness and well-being, including in the neighbourhood context.

Keywords Spirituality · Happiness · Community well-being · Sustainability

---

E. Berejnoi (✉)
311 E Huntington Dr., Tempe, AZ 85282, USA
e-mail: eberejno@asu.edu

R. Ulluwishewa
No 20, Heatley Avenue Hokothitu, Palmerston North 4410, New Zealand
e-mail: ulluwishewa@xtra.co.nz

S. Cloutier
Wrigley Hall, 800 Cady Mall, Tempe, AZ 85281, USA
e-mail: scloutie@asu.edu

L. Gibbons
15 W Buena Vista Dr., Tempe, AZ 85284, USA
e-mail: lvgibbon@asu.edu

S. Puga
922 E Apache Blvd Apt 303, Tempe, AZ 85281, USA
e-mail: spuga@asu.edu

A. Uthumange
Center for Spirituality in Sustainable Business Management, Faculty of Management Studies and Commerce, University of Sri Jayewardenepura, Gangodawila, Sri Lanka
e-mail: uthumange@sjp.ac.lk

© Springer Nature Switzerland AG 2019
Y. Kee et al. (eds.), *Perspectives on Community Well-Being*, Community Quality-of-Life and Well-Being, https://doi.org/10.1007/978-3-030-15115-7_11

11.1 Introduction

There is a growing consensus that happiness and sustainability are interconnected (Brown & Kasser, 2005; Kjell & Candland, 2011; Nisbet, Zelenski, & Murphy, 2011; O'Brien, 2013). Herein, we refer to happiness as subjective well-being or eudaimonia (i.e., cultivation of selflessness and virtue; Joshanloo, 2014), and sustainability as sustainable behaviour which includes measures and practices for a sustainable society. While some studies have provided evidence to show that happy people are more likely to embrace sustainable practices (Brown & Kasser, 2005), other studies have provided evidence to show that those who embrace sustainable practices are likely to be happier (Kasser & Sheldon, 2002; Kellert & Wilson, 1993; O'Brien, 2001). However, the link between sustainability and happiness, and how it contributes to community well-being development, has received little attention from the scientific world.

Our study presented in this chapter is grounded in evidence from quantum physics, neuroscience, transpersonal psychology and studies on consciousness. We identify spirituality as the missing link between happiness and sustainability and point out that as humans grow spiritually, there is are tendencies to become happier and embrace sustainable practices. The following aspects are presented to set the context and perspective of connecting spirituality with happiness and well-being:

- Spirituality is the awareness and experience of belonging to the larger, interconnected community of life, of the purpose and meaning of life within this context, and the development of personal and community values and actions out of these. In other words, spirituality is a process of inner transformation, a transformation from self-centeredness to selflessness, from greed to generosity, from fear to courage, from disharmony to harmony within the self, from fear to love, and from "I" to "we" (Ulluwishewa, 2016). It is a personal transformation within individuals.
- Studies on consciousness describe the experience of spirituality as mindfulness of the present moment. This experience can emerge as a process of self-awareness and self-reflection. The right side of the brain, in charge of creativity, spontaneous communication, and receiving sensory information, plays a big role in staying present (Buck, 1980). The experience of mindfulness can be enhanced by learning to quiet the left side of the brain, which is in charge of logic and thinking. (For particular case studies on consciousness see Alexander, 2012; Alexander & Newell, 2017; Taylor, 2006).
- As we grow spiritually we become happier, peaceful, more loving, more compassionate, wiser and more creative (Zohar, Marshall, & Marshall, 2000). And eventually we become less selfish and more altruistic and act for the well-being of all fellow human beings and their communities, and the natural environment (Horlings, 2015).
- So, as we grow spiritually, we become happier and our intrinsic behaviour becomes more sustainable. However, as discussed later in this study, there are external forces which may also make our behaviour sustainable.

We suggest spirituality to be the ultimate source of both happiness and sustainability. Happiness is a state of mind we experience when we grow spiritually, and sustainability is the behaviour resulting from our spiritual growth. We suggest that individuals are born spiritual beings who, in the process of socialization and acculturalization, lose their spiritual experience. Zohar et al. (2000) state:

> "The self also, we assume, has a source, an origin in the history and development of the universe and a starting point in its own history. Physically, we begin as stardust that has itself evolved out of the quantum vacuum. Spiritually, too, we may begin as proto-consciousness associated with that stardust. As infants, we begin as innocent, undifferentiated consciousness" (p. 125).

The active process of becoming spiritual brings us back closer to our natural spiritual experience. As a personal emergence within individuals, spirituality is affected by both outer and inner circumstances. While the outer circumstances include social, economic and environmental characteristics of the place where the person lives and works, the collective inner existence includes the person's state of mind and culture, and whether the mind is at peace and free from negativities such as greed, anger, hatred, envy and/or anxiety. Therefore, one's spiritual emergence can be accelerated by creating conducive outer circumstances via infrastructural, institutional and technological changes, and by supporting individuals to increase their capacity to extend love to individuals, keep the mind at peace and free from negativities (Krempl, 2014).

This understanding led us to develop a holistic development model that can be used as a guide by those who seek a form of development that is sustainable. At the same time, we propose that our model can aid in delivering higher levels of community well-being and happiness.

11.2 Happiness and Sustainability

This section provides a review of empirical evidence to show the association and interconnectedness between happiness and sustainability.

11.2.1 Happiness Leads to Sustainability

In a study by Brown and Kasser (2005) on happiness and ecological well-being, results reported that participants whose subjective well-being was ruled by intrinsic values (that is, values that come from within) were more inclined toward ecologically responsible behaviour. Mindfulness practices and voluntary simplicity included as part of a eudaimonic lifestyle also related to ecological responsible behaviour. Individuals whose actions are motivated by intrinsic values tend to be less consumerist because they see that excessive material goods do not always add value to their lives, thus, their actions promote sustainable behaviour by having a smaller ecological footprint. In a study on environmental performance in former Soviet countries from 1990 to 2000, Zidanšek (2007) points out that happier nations emit less CO_2 emissions than less happy nations. In fact, happier nations in this study are more energy efficient and produce less CO_2 per unit of GDP. In addition, O'Brien (2012) argues that we are more likely to lead more sustainable lives when we become aware that our pursuit of happiness is interdependent with the happiness of others and that of the environment, this includes our sustainable behaviour. Finally, Cloutier and Pfeiffer (2015) suggest that a sustainable future can be achieved by placing a higher emphasis on measures to enhance community happiness.

11.2.2 Sustainability Leads to Happiness

Activities that promote sustainable behaviour have been proven to lead to happiness. One such activity is the walk to school movement that encourages school children to walk or bike to school (O'Brien, 2001). There is an increase of Safe Routes to School (SRTS) movements worldwide to promote walking to school, which not only promotes sustainable behaviour, but the action of being physically active promotes well-being and satisfaction among participants (O'Brien, 2001). Another study conducted by Kasser and Sheldon (2002), predicted that individuals who engage in environmentally friendly consumption during the holidays tend to experience more happiness. Pursuing a materialistic lifestyle (which does not exemplify sustainable behaviour) results in unhappiness (Richins & Dawson, 1992). This behaviour tends to exist because the individual is motivated by extrinsic goals which do not contribute to finding meaning in life. Sustainable behaviour starts when individuals follow intrinsic goals, which then leads to happiness. Finally, humans are born with an innate need for nature (Kellert & Wilson, 1993), which promotes sustainable behaviour (Conn, 1998), and in turn, increases well-being and happiness (Nisbet et al., 2011). The evidence suggesting that sustainability measures lead to happiness has lead Cloutier, Jambeck, and Scott (2014a) to develop an index for measuring sustainability and happiness for community development. Furthermore, Cloutier, Larson, and Jambeck (2014b) suggest that sustainable development "may function as a driver of residential happiness" (p. 643). In their study on happiness and sustainable development index rankings, they found that two out of the four indexes—Green Cities and Popular Science rankings—were strongly associated with self-reported happiness (Cloutier et al., 2014). Other studies supporting that sustainability leads to happiness both at the individual and community level include Larson et al. (2016), White et al. (2013), Zidanšek (2007), and Zhang, van den Berg, Van Dijk, & Weitkamp (2017).

11.3 Policy Opportunities

The trajectory the world is taking in terms of happiness and sustainability points out that we have come to a point where both these dimensions need to be more connected. As O'Brien (2013), states "The union of sustainability, happiness, and well-being is inevitable, and sustainable happiness has the potential to create game-changing shifts in attitudes, policies, practices, and behaviours" (p. 250). Worldwide organizations are now promoting sustainable initiatives that also promote happiness. The United Nations (UN) is one of the global organizations looking at happiness with a critical eye. Since 2012, the UN has been releasing an annual *World Happiness Report* that explores common variables that can promote happiness at the cross-nation level. The 2018 report points out to five key variables, other than per capita income, to promote well-being: "population health (measured by health-adjusted life expectancy, HALE); the strength of social support networks; personal freedom (measured by the perceived freedom of individuals to make key life decisions); social trust (measured by the public's perception of corruption in government and business); and generosity" (Helliwell, Layard, & Sachs, 2018, p. 150).

What is this information telling us? We propose that it indicates a need for policies that promote happiness and well-being to achieve more sustainable societies starting at the small scale. Happiness should not come at the expense of others or the planet because it would not sustain itself for long. O'Brien (2010) defines sustainable happiness as "happiness that contributes to individual, community and/or global well-being without exploiting other people, the environment or future generations" (n.p.). Thus, to experience sustainable happiness, sustainable behaviour must also enter the game. Examples of policy opportunities include: investing in public libraries in low income neighbourhoods, starting family wellness programs in the community, promoting talks on belonging and mindfulness, encouraging the incorporation of sustainable behaviours (e.g., food gardens, composting, clean energy) at the household and community level and providing incentives (e.g., economic, social, environmental) that will benefit all members of a community.

11.4 Understanding Spirituality, Happiness and Sustainability

In this section, we present perspectives on the three areas of spirituality, happiness, and sustainability and indicate considerations for points of intersection and connection.

11.4.1 Spirit and Spirituality

Spirit is considered by some as the prime energy which gives life to all living and non-living beings. It is conscious, aware and "can think" (Ulluwishewa, 2016, p. 157). This prime energy fills the whole universe. In spite of its vastness, this mass field of energy functions as an indivisible and inseparable single field. From this perspective, the universe is a living being (Capra, 2010). It is known by various names: Universal

Consciousness, Ultimate Truth, Infinite Being, and Higher Self. In most religions, it is personified as God, Allah, Jehovah and Brahman, among others.

The Universal Consciousness, while remaining as an indivisible and inseparable single entity at the quantum level, manifests itself as many material forms (e.g., rocks, soils, plants, animals and human beings). From its perspective, we all are its inseparable parts. Therefore, it feels our pains and pleasures, and we can feel the pains and pleasure of the universe as well (Cozolino, 2014). Hence, we all benefit when everyone is happy, healthy, peaceful, and prosperous. Feeling a state of unity with the universe can be described as unconditional love. This sense of connectedness may be experienced through peace, happiness, wisdom, intelligence and creativity (Cozolino, 2014).

However, we perceive ourselves as separate individuals, as beings separated from others and the natural environment—even ourselves! This perceived separateness is soft-wired in our brain, meaning that our " brain has been programmed by our wrong perceptions to see ourselves, not as integral parts of the whole, but as individuals separate from others and from the environment, and to perceive our fellow human beings as 'others'—competitors and enemies (Ulluwishewa, 2016, p. 162). Therefore, we behave as self-centred individuals. This behavior is culturally learned, driven by mechanisms that have ensured our fitness in the past (Davis, 2017). However, our brain is hard-wired for ethical behaviour and altruism (Cozolino, 2014). Pfaff (2007) suggests four mechanisms that can be mapped in our brain for this intrinsic behaviour: (1) we consider how our actions will affect other people (e.g., throw a rock at somebody), represented in the nervous system; (2) then, mirror neurons are activated when we envision ourselves doing the action; (3) we blur identities of the individuals involved, leading to activation of various brain systems, such as the one related to empathy; and (4) we decide whether to perform the action. A sense of separateness occurs when step 3 is omitted (Pfaff, 2007). When acting under our soft-wired brain, we are inclined to achieve our well-being even at the expense of the well-being of others and the natural environment; yet, we are more likely to behave altruistically toward our social groups (Mathur, Harada, Lipke, & Chiao, 2010). When individuals act under a soft-wired brain of separateness, they do not mind meeting their needs even at the expense of the ability of others and future generations to meet their needs (Dalai Lama XIV, 2014).

There is hope. We, human beings, are endowed with the capacity to overcome the perceived separateness through love (Cacioppo, Bianchi-Demicheli, Hatfield, & Rapson, 2012; Dalai Lama XIV, 2014). To understand what we mean by love, we refer to Fredrickson's (2013) definition: "...love is the momentary upwelling of three tightly interwoven events: first, a sharing of one or more positive emotions between you or another; second, a synchrony between your and the other person's biochemistry and behaviours; and third, a reflected motive to invest in each other's well-being that brings mutual care" (p. 17). In other words, she refers to the experience of love as *positivity resonance*. We expand the described feelings of love to animals, plants, and elements of nature. Love is hardwired in our brain as a tendency to connect with others and serve others selflessly, as altruism and as the golden rule—treat others as you would like others to treat you (Pfaff, 2007). But, the soft-wired separateness and self-centeredness—the culturally conditioned self—prevent us from being guided by the hardwired love. Spirituality is about re-wiring our brain to empower the hardwired love to guide our behaviour and thereby to overcome the separateness (Ulluwishewa, 2018).

Reasoning with our hard-wired brain, it makes sense to suggest that our life mission as human beings is to experience and recognize our oneness with the universe by means of altruism, unconditional love, and spiritual growth.

11.4.2 Happiness

Happiness or subjective well-being is the ultimate goal we all want to achieve in most of our day-to-day activities (Dalai Lama XIV, 2014; Diener, Oishi, & Lucas, 2003; Ford & Mauss, 2014; Johnston et al., 2012; Lyubomirsky et al., 2005). It is usually measured by simply asking people how satisfied they feel with their lives (Diener, Emmons, Larsen, & Griffin, 1985; Lyubomirsky & Lepper, 1999). Subjective well-being is a combined effect of both pleasure and meaning (what we have been referring to as happiness or eudaimonia throughout the paper). Pleasure is a form of short-lived excitement caused by neurochemical reinforcement of an achieved state we enjoy (Huta & Waterman, 2014). We acknowledge pleasure as a component of happiness within academic literature (Huta & Waterman, 2014; Kováč, 2012) but, henceforth, refer to happiness as something more.

The happiness we speak of is the feeling of goodness, well-being, fulfilment and contentment that we experience when we are in full connection with our inner selves—spirit. This is what Aristotle called *Eudaimonia,* which is broadly defined as human flourishing. The proportion of pleasure and happiness in one's level of subjective well-being, therefore, depends on our level of spiritual growth: those who are at lower levels of their spiritual growth mostly seek pleasure, those who are at higher levels mostly seek happiness. Unsustainability arises when we find ourselves locked in the pleasure-seeking arena.

Experiencing happiness requires us to be in connection with the spirit within ourselves, spirit within fellow human beings, and spirit within nature. Hence, those who pursue happiness more than pleasure tend to stay connected to their inner selves, their fellow human beings and nature. They live in alignment with the principle of oneness and follow the golden rule (Block-Lerner et al., 2007; Horlings, 2015).

On the other hand, those who seek pleasure more than eudaimonic happiness are engaged in a continuous struggle of seeking pleasure and avoiding pain. They may find their life somewhat satisfactory in the short-run if they have enough material wealth to continuously experience pleasurable activities. But they struggle to find life satisfaction in the long run. Their unending struggle to earn material wealth leads to disappointments, sorrow, stress, depression and conflictive relationships. They value material wealth, physical pleasure, position, power, social status, and respect more than love, compassion, generosity, tolerance and forgiveness. Evidence suggest that they are highly unlikely to act for the well-being of others and the natural environment (Zylstra, Knight, Esler, & Le Grange, 2014).

11.4.3 Sustainability

Sustainability is popularly defined as meeting the needs of the present generation without compromising the needs of future generations (Brundtland et al., 1987). Implicit in this definition are concepts of intragenerational justice and externalities, among others; yet, under this definition, these issues are primarily focused on one dimension of sustainability—the temporal dimension, which looks at "sustainability over time and bringing justice to future generations" (p. 66).

This definition does not explicitly recognize the possibility of meeting the needs of one community or one country at the expense of the ability of another community or another country to meet their needs. It is important to raise awareness of the interconnected and interdependent world we live in today, and, to place higher emphasis on working toward sustainability in every region in the world. Many countries and regions in the world meet their needs at the expense of communities and countries under their domination. Yet, this is neither sustainable in the long term nor ethical.

We propose Uluwishewa's (2018) definition which accommodates both temporal and spatial dimensions of sustainability: "Sustainability is the ability of any individual, community or country to meet their needs and live happily without compromising the ability of other individuals, communities, countries and future generations to meet their needs and live happily" (p. 66).

The human society consists of many communities and many countries. If any community/country meets its needs at the expense of the ability of another community/country to meet their needs, the human society cannot be sustainable. If we think of the tragedy of the commons, when everybody takes resources without mindfully leaving some for the future, at some point, we will run out of resources. In this case, acting with a mindful and altruistic heart, also means being smart about managing our resources across space and time.

11.5 Spirituality: The Missing Link

Perhaps the best way to discover the third factor which links happiness and sustainability is to discover the root causes of unhappiness and unsustainability we are witnessing across the world. If we find that unsustainability and unhappiness are caused by the same factor, that factor could be the one linking sustainability and happiness. This section takes a deep look into unsustainability and unhappiness we are witnessing in our societies today in order to discover their root causes.

11.5.1 Why "Unsustainability"?

One's behaviour in sustainable lifestyle demands pursuit of the well-being for oneself, others, and the natural environment equally. Why can't we treat equally ourselves, others, and nature?

- We are soft-wired with a false perception of separateness. Joshanloo (2014) states: "perceiving the self as separate from the non-self leads to unnecessary personal desires, and these desired are blamed for causing suffering. In order to stop the suffering, one needs to achieve a state of inner peace by realizing that the separation of the self and the non-self is but an illusion" (p. 479).
- We experience cravings and aversions. Each and every one of us has a unique set of cravings and aversions which make us pleasure-seekers and pain-avoiders, leading the way to greed, discomfort, and suffering (Chen, 2006). In fact, the Dalai Lama XIV (2014) states:

> "Whatever material comforts we have, we are still afflicted by greed, jealousy, and competitiveness. As long as these disturbing emotions remain intact, we continue to experience suffering. Besides which, when the focus is solely on material development, there does not seem to be much need for love and compassion. For example, we do not need love and compassion to develop new machinery. Therefore, if human beings think only about their physical problems and try to counter them in exclusively material ways, they will naturally ignore such inner values as loving-kindness and compassion. Indeed, two centuries of scientific and technological development have inclined people in many parts of the world to consider material prosperity to be of greater worth than inner qualities" (p. 6).

- When we are indulged in a pleasurable experience, depending on our attachment to the experience, we will want to prolong the period of the pleasure-experience at any cost, even at the expense of our own long-term well-being, the well-being of others and the natural environment (Dalai Lama XIV, 2014; Zylstra et al., 2014). Research has shown, however, that we aren't very good at understanding when an activity is no longer providing us happiness (Lyubomirsky et al., 2005; Nesse, 2004). We stay invested in similar activities for long periods of time.
- Individuals, corporations, and governments (political leaders) oftentimes seek the pleasure of getting power, higher profits, higher social status, and respect. Hence, they fail to see the long-term consequences of their short-sighted decisions for themselves, others and nature. This failure to foretell how our actions will affect the future may be caused by a naïve lack of understanding of the interrelationship between their actions and future trade-offs, or by an egotistical position to not consider the affected populations.
- Consequently, we all become more self-centred and more unsustainable in our behaviour.
- Conversely, there is also the case of unsustainability caused by lack of access to education and resources. Much global unsustainable behaviour is done to survive. Other individuals, for example, may have access to resources, yet lack a critical understanding of the environmental impacts they may cause with their action and behaviours.

11.5.2 Why Unhappiness?

Happiness is, as demonstrated above, an attribute of Spirit. We can experience it only when we strive to become one with spirit or become spiritual. How does a person become one with the spirit and become happy?

- Spirit lies within us, in others and in nature.
- Becoming one with spirit means connecting to the spirit within us, within others and within nature.
- Connecting means not only physical nearness, touch and likeness, but also unselfish interaction. For example:
  - Spirit within us: What keeps us separated from the spirit within us is our sense of 'I'/Ego which acts for 'my' pleasure at the expense of my own long-term well-being, the well-being of others and the well-being of nature. The notion of I/ego is a product of the soft-wired brain, and the neuroplasticity of the brain allows us to change the soft-wired brain permanently. However, this is far from reality in our ordinary life. In our ordinary life, our notion of I/ego becomes weak and is temporarily dissolved when we are in deep meditation/prayer or when we are in a state of peace or when we are deeply engaged in any action, (e.g., reading, singing or teaching). On the other hand, it becomes strong when we are agitated, when we are challenged or threatened. We become one with the spirit within when the notion of 'I'/Ego is transcended by the individual's higher consciousness. Then, we connect with the spirit within and experience happiness.
  - Spirit within others: When we interact with others without the sense of 'I'/Ego, we see them without prejudices and judgements, and we collaborate with them without expecting anything in return. We also see our understanding of others as only a reflection of ourselves. Then we connect with their inner selves, the spirit within and experience happiness.
  - Spirit within nature: Seeing the beauty of nature without becoming attached to its commercial value; seeing nature with the attitude of gratitude for giving us life (e.g., oxygen and food); caring for nature and nurturing it; seeing nature without wanting to possess it or without wanting to gain some selfish benefits from it. If we interact with nature like this, we will directly connect with the spirit and experience peace and happiness.

Yet, most of us, especially in the West, are not in contact with the spirit within us, or interact with others and nature with self-centred interests in mind. Zohar, Marshall, and Marshall (2000) add "Western culture is ego-dominated. Its emphasis is on public personas and formal relationships, and its extreme emphasis is on the isolated individual who must constantly make rational decisions. This is why most of us in the West live from the periphery of ourselves, wrongly believing ego to be the whole story of the self" (p. 128). Hence, we fail to experience happiness. Thus, we suggest our spiritual underdevelopment to be the root cause of our unhappiness.

11.6 The Missing Link

We have provided evidence that the same factor may cause both unsustainability and unhappiness: it is our spiritual underdevelopment. Therefore, spirituality must be the missing link between sustainability and happiness. As we grow spiritually, we stay in touch with the spirit within us, with the spirit within our fellow human beings, and with the spirit within the natural environment during most of our waking life, and therefore we lead the way to more intrinsic happiness and sustainable behaviour.

When intrinsically connected within and outside us, sustainable behaviour is our default behaviour and happiness is our default feeling. Spirituality is the key to unlock happiness and sustainable behaviours hidden within us.

11.7 Towards a Framework for Holistic Development

As already seen, the purpose of our life as human beings is to grow spiritually—transcending our illusionary perception of separateness and realizing our oneness with fellow human beings and nature—which provides access to peace, happiness, wisdom, creativity and intelligence hidden within us. If any form of development is to be holistic, it must be aligned with the purpose. Such a form of development contributes not only to the physical quality of life but also to spiritual growth, which eventually makes people happy and their behaviour sustainable.

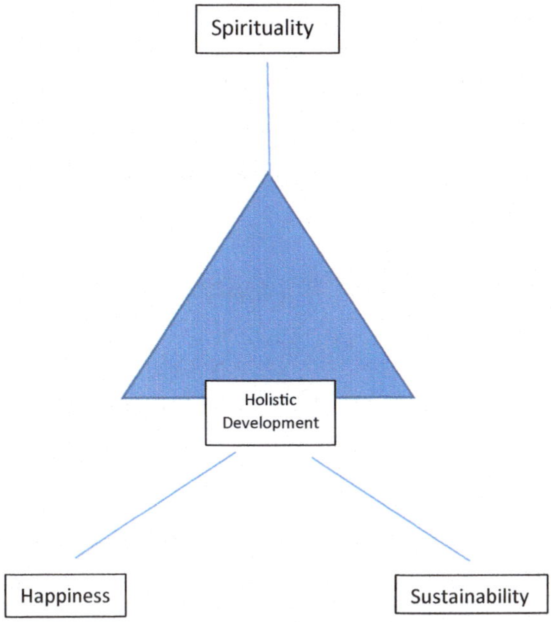

As individuals grow spiritually, they become happier and behave in a sustainable way. While spirituality is the cause, happiness and sustainability are its effects. However, studies on happiness and sustainability show many other ways to make people happy and promote sustainability. For instance, while providing better amenities and more recreation facilities, raising income, providing access to open spaces and greeneries, and providing more opportunities to connect with others are recommended to enhance happiness, providing technological, infrastructural and institutional infrastructures conducive to sustainability are also recommended to work toward a more sustainable future. The extrinsic measures described above are necessary in the fast-changing world we live in, but they by themselves are not enough to permanently remove the root cause of growing unhappiness and unsustainability: the sense of separateness soft-wired in our brain and resulting self-centeredness, greed, and fears. Only spiritual growth in individuals can do it. We present the following points of perspective to consider about holistic development:

- What we call sustainable development today is not holistic and hence fails to be sustainable and deliver happiness. As previously discussed in the paper, a more holistic view of sustainable development would include both a special and temporal scale to this definition.
- We cannot expect governments, international agencies, and corporations to lead holistic development. In fact, holistic development can arise only from an intrinsic motivation from ordinary people at the grassroots level.
- The proportion of the world's population living in cities is on the rise. The World Health Organization (WHO) (2015) reports that in 2015, 54% of the global population lived in urban areas, an increase of 30% from 1950. Estimates show that this rate will continue increasing approximately 1.84% per year between 2015 and 2020, reaching 60% of the world population living in urban areas by 2030 (WHO, 2015). Hence, holistic development should arise as urban neighbourhoods-based community development projects.
- This study is an attempt to develop a framework for holistic development that can be used as a guide for such urban neighbourhood-based holistic development.

11.8 Unsustainability and Unhappiness in Urban Neighbourhoods

Further, there are other perspectives to consider, including for neighbourhoods, in the context of unsustainability and unhappiness. These are:

- The root cause of continuing unhappiness is our perceived separateness between 'I'/self, others, and nature.
- The separateness is a more serious issue in cities than in country sides and rural areas (Knight & Gunatilaka, 2010; Tonkiss, 2005; Young, Diep, & Drabble, 2006). Tonkiss (2005) discusses the human disconnection created by the modern city, caused by separation of physical space and by a place filled with strangers. He

states that disconnect from others is a social norm in the city, and that following the status quo ensures peace and order. We also add that the sense of separateness creates feelings of exclusion and othering.

- The separateness reflects outwardly as breaking down of families and communities. That is why social disconnectedness, alienation, and loneliness have become serious social issues.
- Consumerism rampant in urban society strengthens separateness. How?
  - Separateness is strengthened by the differences in likes and dislikes of individuals. Attachment to *likes* leads to craving, and attachment to *dislikes* leads to aversion; each and every person has a unique set of cravings and aversions which strengthens separateness from others and the natural environment. In a simplistic example, when a person is attached to a craving, they may behave in ways to have more of that particular object/service which in turn, would strengthen the craving. This can lead the person to focus on their personal cravings rather than to the needs of others (which includes the environment). Thus, strong attachments make us less receptive to altruism and to an inner connection with ourselves.
  - Consumerism feeds cravings—the more we have, the more attached we are to material possessions, and the stronger the craving for consumption.
  - Consumerism creates unique sets of cravings (and aversions) in each age/gender group such as children, adolescents, teenagers, youths, middle-agers, and elderly people. Each group has its own unique set of cravings and aversions.
  - The uniqueness of their cravings and aversions makes it difficult for each group to share their resources with other groups within family as well as within community. This encourages separateness. For instance, in the same family, children, adolescents, and parents cannot share the same TV, same food, same family phone; young children tend to leave parents and live separately, parents send grandparents to elderly homes.
  - Growing separateness causes unhappiness and unsustainability in Western cities and neighbourhoods where consumerism is dominant (Berry & Okulicz-Kozaryn, 2011). According to research conducted by Berry and Okulicz-Kozaryn (2011), this situation is more prevalent in Western countries, or in countries that use a Western European foundation, where happiness decreases as we move from rural communities to urbanized and large cities.
  - Growing separateness increases competition between individuals, leading to feelings of "us better than them," leading way to conflict.
  - However, the growing separateness and resulting unhappiness and unsustainability generates market for more goods and services which promote business, increase profit and GDP.

11.9 How to Achieve Holistic Development in Urban Neighbourhoods?

Human beings are endowed with the capacity to overcome the separateness by *love* and thereby to achieve *oneness* and make the world a happy, peaceful and prosperous place. By *oneness*, we refer to an intrinsic connection that humans feel with the rest of humanity via the experience of love. When *I* feel unconditional love toward others, I will no longer be *I*, but *we*. The feeling of oneness emerges as love is cultivated. The outcome from love and oneness is a prosperous society, one where mindfulness and cooperation are what drive people, rather than competition and greed. What can people in neighbourhoods do to achieve such a state?

In the first place, it is important to be aware of two types of separateness: (1) Inner Separateness: it refers to a mind-body disconnect, which is invisible to the eye, but visible to the intuition and can be measured through rigorous scientific procedures (Daubenmier, Sze, Kerr, Kemeny, & Mehling, 2013; Frewen & Lanius, 2006; Saunders et al., 2007). Inner separateness may arise due to an overemphasis on the external environment, a drive for competition, and hardship to make ends meet, among many other causes. (2) Outer Separateness: it refers to social disconnectedness and alienation, oftentimes experienced in urban societies.

11.9.1 To Overcome Inner Separateness

- Engage in activities that create a mind-body connection. An example of such an activity is brain-heart coherence researched by the HeartMath Institute (McCraty, 2015; McCraty, Atkinson, Tomasino, & Bradley, 2009). The activity takes three steps: (1) shift focus from the brain to the heart. (2) breath in and out as slow as possible. Breathing slowly is a sign of safety. We can trigger the mind and heart to feel safer by breathing at a slow pace. (3) feel gratitude, appreciation, kindness, and forgiveness from the heart. Doing this activity for three minutes has proven to have an effect in the individual for as long as six hours after the activity was performed (Braden, 2017).
- Engage in meditation and mindfulness practices (see Dalai Lama XIV, 2014; Nidich et al., 2009; Salzberg, 2010; Wallace & Shapiro, 2006; Wamsler et al., 2018; Zeidan, Diamond, & Goolkasian, 2010).
- Engage in a gratitude practice (e.g., via journaling, poetry, group talk). Experiments demonstrate that a gratitude practice increases positive affect, mood and well-being (Watkins, Woodward, Stone, & Kolts, 2003), improves quality of sleep (Emmons, McCullough, & Diener, 2003), decreases depressive symptoms (Krause, 2009), and enhances pro-social behaviour (Bartlett & Desteno, 2006).
- Provide facilities to develop spiritual knowledge and understanding. For instance, a community spiritual center that provides spiritual talks, seminars, discussions,

yoga, spiritual therapy and spiritual-based music, sports, games, meditation and a community library with spiritual literature.
- Provide facilities to use the spiritual knowledge and understanding to overcome inner separateness. For instance, organizing spiritual-based service activities (e.g., helping others without expecting anything in return). Taking part in such activities reduces self-centeredness, which eventually overcomes inner separateness. The human brain is soft wired (in a self-centred way) to make others expect benefits to the self. Helping others without expecting any self-benefit will re-wire our brain to reduce our self-centeredness. Then we begin to enjoy the happiness of giving more than the happiness of receiving and accumulating.

11.9.2 To Overcome Outer Separateness

- Form community/neighbourhood organizations.
- Hold dialogs/discussions in organizations to identify the root cause of unhappiness and unsustainability as the separateness, and measures to overcome the separateness.
- Provide more opportunities for individuals to meet and interact with each other, and to enhance the level of happiness and sustainability of the neighbourhood. In identifying measures/projects, the goal should aim at overcoming separateness rather than enhancing happiness and sustainability. The reason for this is that some individuals may come up with measures and/or projects which enhance happiness and/or sustainability but further strengthen separateness. Some sample measures/projects for overcoming outer separateness (from others and from nature) while promoting happiness and sustainability are: improving walkability, encouraging cycling and the use of public transport, establishing public parks and open spaces, providing more public recreation facilities and amenities, organizing community festivals and activities such as sports, music, dancing, etc.
- Provide more opportunities to connect and interact with nature. This can be done by incorporating natural processes in the community and making them more visible, such as restoring urban streams, developing urban gardens and CSA's, and incorporating composting programs.
- Identify income-generating opportunities which promote/do not conflict with outer and inner connectedness.

As the activities help to overcome both inner and outer separateness, people grow spiritually and eventually become happier and behave in sustainable ways. While the inner connectedness contributes to the outer connectedness, the outer connectedness contributes to the inner connectedness. Inner and outer measures should take place simultaneously for more effective and lasting change in the community. The graph below indicates how the process of holistic development emerges.

11.10 Outline of the Framework for Holistic Development

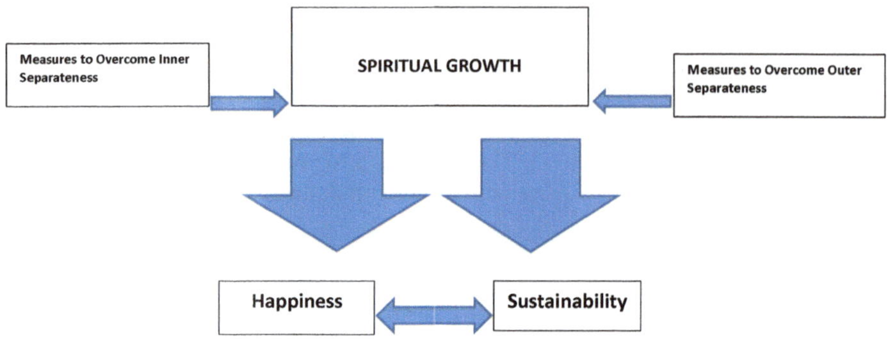

The measures adopted to overcome inner and outer connectedness have the potential to create lasting results in a community when applied simultaneously. Spiritual growth takes place when there is a process for both inner and outer connectedness. As the individual grows spiritually, they become more mindful toward their actions as well as more reflective on how their thoughts, behaviours, and actions have an effect on the wider ecosystem. With more mindfulness in our actions, there is an intrinsic desire to behave sustainably, and by behaving in such a way, we feel genuine happiness because we feel connected at a deeper level with existence and our actions speak love.

Therefore, holistic development considers spirituality as its core. The model provides a guide for community members, grassroots organizations, policy makers, and planners to set goals and to identify projects and strategies for holistic development. The model suggests two sets of projects:

(1) projects which provide physical infrastructural facilities, institutional strategies and technologies that are necessary for individuals to overcome their existing separateness from others and from natural environment.
(2) projects which provide facilities for individuals to gain spiritual understanding.

The model emphasizes the significance of having projects and activities aimed at all three goals: growing spiritually, enhancing happiness, and working toward sustainability. It also emphasizes the significance of ensuring the harmony among the activities performed. For instance, the activities undertaken for enhancing happiness should not conflict with those undertaken for achieving sustainability and promoting spiritual growth. Likewise, the activities undertaken for spiritual growth should not conflict with happiness and sustainability.

11.11 Conclusion

This chapter provides an exploration of what we call the missing link between happiness and sustainability. Through an extensive evaluation of the connection between happiness and sustainability and the causes of unhappiness and unsustainability, we suggest that the missing link is spirituality. We presented spirituality in rational and scientific terms and defined it as the experience to belonging to the larger living and non-living ecosystem. The process of spiritual growth allows individuals to become mindful of their thoughts, actions, and behaviour, leading to happier and more sustainable communities. Gutenschwager (2013) points out that the development of altruistic societies starts at the local level, creating a rippling effect to the larger scale. It is through the process of spiritual emergence that we become more altruistic and consider the well-being of everyone in the temporal and spatial scales.

We have provided a framework for individuals and neighbourhoods to achieve lasting happiness and sustainability by mindfully working on the following processes:

(1) Inner connectedness: Engage in spiritual practices to reconnect within and facilitate this process to other individuals.
(2) Outer connectedness: Incorporate educational, infrastructural, institutional, and technological measures at the community level to reconnect as a community and as part of the ecosystem.

Using this framework, we suggest that while the inner connectedness contributes to the outer connectedness, the outer connectedness contributes to inner connectedness.

The measures adopted for outer connectedness can generate a superficial connectedness with others and with nature, but there is no intrinsic inner connectedness (e.g., selfless relationships, connection with the spirit within others and within nature). The outer connectedness is self-centred. Such a superficial connectedness can overcome the pain/suffering caused by existing disconnectedness/loneliness and make people feel pleasure (or hedonic happiness). But without the inner connectedness with the spirit within others and within nature which generates happiness, people cannot experience true happiness. Most community-based projects aimed at happiness and sustainability (without spirituality) fail to deliver "true" happiness and achieve "true" sustainability. In such projects, only those who are in the process of spiritual growth would experience "true" happiness and effortlessly behave in sustainable ways (voluntarily embrace sustainable practices).

However, such an outer connectedness facilitates inner connectedness. Positive interactions with others and with nature re-wires our brains and prepares us for inner connectedness. Those who interact negatively will not experience this. Most people find it hard to achieve spiritual growth first. Hence, it is wise to adopt measures necessary for the second endeavour. Community development programmes can create an environment conducive to outer connectedness which will eventually help people achieve inner connectedness. The resulting inner and outer connectedness will lead to a lasting experience of happiness and sustainability.

References

Alexander, E. (2012). *Proof of heaven: A neurosurgeon's journey into the afterlife*. New York: Simon and Schuster.

Alexander, E., & Newell, K. (2017). *Living in a mindful universe: A neurosurgeon's journey into the heart of consciousness* [Kindle Version]. Retrieved from amazon.com.

Bartlett, M., & Desteno, D. (2006). Gratitude and prosocial behavior: Helping when it costs you. *Psychological Science, 17*(4), 319–325.

Berry, B., & Okulicz-Kozaryn, A. (2011). An urban-rural happiness gradient. *Urban Geography, 32*(6), 871–883.

Block-Lerner, J., Adair, C., Plumb, J., Rhatigan, D., & Orsillo, S. (2007). The case for mindfulness-based approaches in the cultivation of empathy: Does nonjudgmental, present-moment awareness increase capacity for perspective-taking and empathic concern? *Journal of Marital and Family Therapy, 33*(4), 501–516.

Braden, G. (2017). Awakening the heart-brain union. In *Missing links*. Gaia TV.

Brown, K., & Kasser, T. (2005). Are psychological and ecological well-being compatible? The role of values, mindfulness and lifestyle. *Social Indicators Research, 74*, 349–368.

Brundtland, G., Khalid, M., Agnelli, S., Al-Athel, S., Chidzero, B., Fadika, L., ... Singh, M. (1987). Our common future (\'brundtland report\').

Buck, R. (1980). *Left and right hemisphere brain functions and symbolic vs. spontaneous communication processes*. S.I.: Distributed by ERIC Clearinghouse.

Cacioppo, S., Bianchi-Demicheli, F., Hatfield, E., & Rapson, R. L. (2012). Social neuroscience of love. *Clinical Neuropsychiatry, 9*(1).

Capra, F. (2010). *The Tao of physics: An exploration of the parallels between modern physics and eastern mysticism*. Shambhala Publications.

Chen, Y. H. (2006). Coping with suffering: The Buddhist perspective. In P. T. P. Wong & L. C. J. Wong (Eds.), *Handbook of multicultural perspectives on stress and coping* (pp. 73–89). Dallas, TX: Spring Publications.

Cloutier, S., & Pfeiffer, D. (2015). Sustainability through happiness: A framework for sustainable development. *Sustainable Development, 23*(5), 317–327.

Cloutier, Jambeck, & Scott. (2014a). The sustainable neighborhoods for happiness index (SNHI): A metric for assessing a community's sustainability and potential influence on happiness. *Ecological Indicators, 40*(C), 147–152.

Cloutier, S., Larson, L., & Jambeck, J. (2014b). Are sustainable cities "happy" cities? Associations between sustainable development and human well-being in urban areas of the United States. *Environment, Development and Sustainability, 16*(3), 633–647.

Conn, S. (1998). Living in the earth: Ecopsychology, health and psychotherapy. *The Humanistic Psychologist, 26*, 179–198.

Cozolino, L. (2014). *The neuroscience of human relationships: Attachment and the developing social brain*. WW Norton & Company.

Dalai Lama XIV. (2014). Happiness from a Buddhist perspective. *The Journal of Law and Religion, 29*(1), 5–13.

Daubenmier, J., Sze, J., Kerr, C., Kemeny, M., & Mehling, W. (2013). Follow your breath: Respiratory interoceptive accuracy in experienced meditators. *Psychophysiology, 50*(8), 777–789.

Davis, N. (2017). *The selfish gene*. Macat Library.

Diener, E., Emmons, R., Larsen, R., & Griffin, S. (1985). The satisfaction with life scale. *Journal of Personality Assessment, 49*(1), 71–75.

Diener, E., Oishi, S., & Lucas, R. (2003). Personality, culture, and subjective well-being: Emotional and cognitive evaluations of life. *Annual Review of Psychology, 54*(1), 403–425.

Emmons, R., McCullough, M., & Diener (Ed.). (2003). Counting blessings versus burdens: An experimental investigation of gratitude and subjective well-being in daily life. *Journal of Personality and Social Psychology, 84*(2), 377–389.

Ford, B., & Mauss, I. (2014). The paradoxical effects of pursuing positive emotion: When and why wanting to feel happy backfires. In *Positive emotion* (p. Positive Emotion, Chapter 20). Oxford University Press.

Fredrickson, B. (2013). *Love 2.0*. New York: Penguin Group.

Frewen, P. A., & Lanius, R. A. (2006). Neurobiology of dissociation: Unity and disunity in mind—body–brain. *Psychiatric Clinics, 29*(1), 113–128.

Gutenschwager, G. (2013). From Epicurus to Maslow: Happiness then and now and the place of the human being in social theory. *Cadmus, 1*(6), 66–90.

Helliwell, J., Layard, R., & Sachs, J. D. (2018). *World Happiness Report*.

Horlings, L. (2015). The inner dimension of sustainability: Personal and cultural values. *Current Opinion in Environmental Sustainability, 14,* 163–169.

Huta, V., & Waterman, A. (2014). Eudaimonia and its distinction from Hedonia: Developing a classification and terminology for understanding conceptual and operational definitions. *Journal of Happiness Studies, 15*(6), 1425–1456.

Johnston, B., Colson, E., Falk, D., St John, G., Bodley, J., McCay, B., … Slyomovics, S. (2012). On happiness. *American Anthropologist, 114*(1), 6–18.

Joshanloo, M. (2014). Eastern conceptualizations of happiness: Fundamental differences with western views. *Journal of Happiness Studies, 15*(2), 475–493.

Kasser, T., & Sheldon, K. (2002). What makes for a merry Christmas? *Journal of Happiness Studies*, 313–329.

Keith, (2005). Pursuing happiness: The architecture of sustainable change. *Review of General Psychology, 9*(2), 111–131.

Kellert, S. R., & Wilson, E. O. (Eds.). (1993). *The biophilia hypothesis*. Washington, DC: Island Press.

Kiefer, A., Cloutier, S., & Prosser. (2017). *Community and composting in victory acres*. Arizona State University.

Kjell, O., & Candland, D. K. (2011). Sustainable well-being: A potential synergy between sustainability and well-being research. *Review of General Psychology, 15*(3), 255–266.

Knight and Gunatilaka. (2010). Great expectations? The subjective well-being of rural-urban migrants in China. *World Development, 38*(1), 113–124.

Kováč, L. (2012). The biology of happiness. *EMBO Reports, 13*(4), 297–302.

Krause, N. (2009). Religious involvement, gratitude, and change in depressive symptoms over time. *International Journal for the Psychology of Religion, 19*(3), 155–172.

Krempl, S. (2014). Is spirituality the essence of sustainability? In *The truth is out there* (pp. 169–181). Black Swan Press.

Larson, Keith, Fernandez, Hallo, Shafer, & Jennings. (2016). Ecosystem services and urban greenways: What's the public's perspective? *Ecosystem Services, 22,* 111–116.

Lyubomirsky, S., & Lepper, H. S. (1999). A measure of subjective happiness: Preliminary reliability and construct validation. *Social Indicators Research, 46,* 137–155.

Lyubomirsky, S., Sheldon, K., Schkade, D., Candland, D. K., Baumeister, R. F., & Simonton, D.

Mathur, Harada, Lipke, & Chiao. (2010). Neural basis of extraordinary empathy and altruistic motivation. *NeuroImage, 51*(4), 1468–1475.

McCraty, R. (2015). *Heart-brain neurodynamics: The making of emotions*. HeartMath Institute. Retrieved from https://www.heartmath.org/assets/uploads/2015/03/heart-brain-neurodynamics.pdf.

McCraty, R., Atkinson, M., Tomasino, D., & Bradley, R. T. (2009). The coherent heart heart-brain interactions, psychophysiological coherence, and the emergence of system-wide order. *Integral Review: A Transdisciplinary & Transcultural Journal for New Thought, Research, & Praxis, 5*(2).

Moody, R. (1987). *Life after life: The investigation of a phenomenon, survival of bodily death* (1st large print ed.). New York, NY: Phoenix Press.

Nesse, R. M. (2004). Natural selection and the elusiveness of happiness. *Philosophical Transactions of the Royal Society of London. Series B: Biological Sciences, 359*(1449), 1333–1347. https://doi.org/10.1098/rstb.2004.1511.

Nidich, S., Rainforth, M., Haaga, D., Hagelin, J., Salerno, J., Travis, F., … Schneider, R. (2009). A randomized controlled trial on effects of the transcendental meditation program on blood pressure, psychological distress, and coping in young adults. *American Journal of Hypertension, 22*(12), 1326–1331.

Nisbet, E., Zelenski, J., & Murphy, S. (2011). Happiness is in our nature: Exploring nature relatedness as a contributor to subjective well-being. *Journal of Happiness Studies, 12,* 303–322.

O'Brien, C. (2001). *Ontario walkability study, trip to school: Children's experiences and aspirations*. York University, Canada, York Centre for Applied Sustainability. Retrieved June 28, 2018, from http://ontarioactiveschooltravel.ca/?p__relatedresearch.

O'Brien, C. (2010). Sustainability, happiness and education. *Journal of Sustainability Education, 1*. Retrieved from www.jsedimensions.org/wordpress/content/2010/04/.

O'Brien, C. (2012). Sustainable happiness and well-being: Future directions for positive psychology. *Psychology, 3*(12), 1196.

O'Brien, C. (2013). Happiness and sustainability together at last! Sustainable Happiness. *Canadian Journal of Education, 36*(4), 228–256.

Pfaff, D. (2007). *The neuroscience of fair play: Why we (usually) follow the Golden rule*. New York: Dana Press.

Pfeiffer, D., & Cloutier, S. (2016). Planning for happy neighbourhoods. *Journal of the American Planning Association, 82*(3), 267–279.

Richins, M., & Dawson, S. (1992). A consumer values orientation for materialism and its measurement: Scale development and validation. *Journal of Consumer Research, 19,* 303–316.

Salzberg, S. (2010). *Real happiness: The power of meditation: A 28-day program*. Workman Publishing.

Saunders, P., Tractenberg, R., Chaterji, R., Amri, H., Harazduk, N., Gordon, J., … Haramati, A. (2007). Promoting self-awareness and reflection through an experiential mind-body skills course for first year medical students. *Medical Teacher, 29*(8), 778–784.

Taylor, J. B. (2006). *My stroke of insight: a brain scientist's personal journey*. New York: Plume.

Tonkiss, F. (2005). *Space, the city and social theory: Social relations and urban forms*. Polity.

Ulluwishewa, R. (2016) Spirituality, sustainability and happiness: A quantum-neuroscientific perspective. In: S. Dhiman, J. Marques (Eds.), *Spirituality and sustainability*. Cham: Springer. https://doi.org/10.1007/978-3-319-34235-1_10.

Ulluwishewa, R. (2018). Spirituality, universal love and sustainable behaviour. *Annals of Behavioral Neuroscience, 1*(1), 66–76. ISSN 2638-9231.

Wallace, B. A., & Shapiro, S. L. (2006). Mental balance and well-being: Building bridges between buddhism and western psychology. *American Psychologist, 61*(7), 690–701. https://doi.org/10.1037/0003-066X.61.7.690.

Wamsler, C., Brossmann, J., Hendersson, H., Kristjansdottir, R., Mcdonald, C., & Scarampi, P. (2018). Mindfulness in sustainability science, practice, and teaching. *Sustainability Science, 13*(1), 143.

Watkins, P., Woodward, K., Stone, T., & Kolts, R. (2003). Gratitude and happiness: Development of a measure of gratitude, and relationships with subjective well-being. *Social Behavior and Personality, 31*(5), 431–451.

World Health Organization (WHO). (2015). *Urban population growth*. Retrieved October 18, 2018, from http://www.who.int/gho/urban_health/situation_trends/urban_population_growth/en/index1.html.

Young, C., Diep, M., & Drabble, S. (2006). Living with difference? The 'Cosmopolitan City' and urban reimaging in Manchester, UK. *Urban Studies, 43*(10), 1687–1714.

Zeidan, J., Diamond, D., & Goolkasian, (2010). Mindfulness meditation improves cognition: Evidence of brief mental training. *Consciousness and Cognition, 19*(2), 597–605.

Zhang, Y., van den Berg, A. E., Van Dijk, T., & Weitkamp, G. (2017). Towards Well-being, Innovation Spatial Transformation, and Urban Regional Studies Institute. Quality over quantity: Contribution of urban green space to neighborhood satisfaction. *International Journal of Environmental Research and Public Health, 14*(5), 1661–7827.

Zidanšek, A. (2007). Sustainable development and happiness in nations. *Energy, 32*(6), 891–897.

Zohar, D., Marshall, I., & Marshall, I. N. (2000). *SQ: Connecting with our spiritual intelligence*. USA: Bloomsbury Publishing.

Zylstra, M. J., Knight, A. T., Esler, K. J., & Le Grange, L. L. (2014). Connectedness as a core conservation concern: An interdisciplinary review of theory and a call for practice. *Springer Science Reviews, 2*(1–2), 119–143. https://doi.org/10.1007/s40362-014-0021-3.

Erica Berejnoi Bejarano is a doctoral student in the School of Sustainability as well as a member of the Sustainability & Happiness Research Lab at Arizona State University, whose research includes inner sustainability, spirituality, contemplative practices, happiness, and community development and empowerment. She has published the self-help book *My Gratitude Journal: 30-Day Challenge* and has other writing projects in the works to promote the cultivation of inner sustainability. Erica has a BS in Business Administration and a BA in Asian Studies from Berea College. In addition to her academic endeavors, Erica is a spiritual practitioner, dancer, animal lover, and aspiring professional writer.

Rohana Ulluwishewa is a visiting Professor at the Center for Spirituality in Sustainable Business Management at the University of Sri Jayewardenepura, Sri Lanka. He holds BA Hons. (USJP), M.Sc. (London School of Economics), and a Ph.D. from Kyushu University. In his thirty years of academic career, he has worked as Associate Professor at the University of Sri Jayewardenepura, as Senior Lecturer at the University of Brunei Darussalam, and was a Visiting Fellow at Wageningen Agricultural University in the Netherlands, Leeds University in UK, Leiden University in the Netherlands, and Massey University in New Zealand. He has served as a consultant for numerous national and international development agencies and has published in numerous international journals. For the last decade, the focus of his research and publications has been on spirituality and sustainability. His first book, *Spirituality and Sustainable Development,* was honored as a Finalist of the International Book Award 2014. The second book, *Spirituality Demystified: Understanding Spirituality in Rational Terms,* won the AWCT awards (the highest prize annually awarded in New Zealand for books on Body, Mind and Spirit) in 2015.

Scott Cloutier is an Assistant Professor in the School of Sustainability at Arizona State University. His applied research projects and service-based classes focus on simultaneously promoting greater opportunities for happiness and sustainability. He has experience in community development processes and projects in many locations throughout the United States, on the Navajo and Hopi Reservations in Arizona, in Guatemala, Mexico, Denmark, Costa Rica, and Bolivia. Ultimately, he strives to be deeply humble, open-minded, and open-hearted, while drawing on his experiences and skills as a US veteran, engineer, scientist, and scholar to serve a brighter future.

Leah V. Gibbons is a scholar, practitioner, and teacher of ecological, sustainable design and development. Her focus is on regenerative development and design. She works with communities at all scales to co-create continually higher levels of health and vitality. As a scholar, Leah's work involves examining how socio-ecological (i.e., living) systems can be designed, planned, and developed to be optimally healthy for all life and to catalyze vitality across scales. Her research addresses two themes: 1. shifts in consciousness to a holistic worldview and 2. shifts in development and design outcomes that enable increasing systemic health and vitality. Within these two themes, she examines what common success factors, challenges, and approaches to overcome challenges are. She uses mixed-method approaches in both natural and social sciences to create transferable, actionable knowledge bridging the knowledge-action gap in sustainability, design, planning, and development. Leah is Principal and Founder at Koru Collaborative, an ecological and regenerative development and design firm. This role builds on her 20+ years of experience and expertise in the fields of sustainability consulting, green and natural building, landscape design, restoration ecology, invasion biology, and holistic health coaching. Leah's work is supported by her Doctoral candidacy in Sustainability from Arizona University; a MS in Ecology and Evolutionary Biology from The University of Tennessee, with a focus on community ecology and invasion biology; a BS in Biology and Anthropology from Vanderbilt University, with a focus on human-nature interactions; and her professional practice integrating science, design, and their theoretical and practical outcomes.

Susana Puga is an undergraduate studying Sustainability at Arizona State University. Susie is currently working as a garden instructor at Broadmor Elementary School where she is able to reach over 800 children with environmental science education. Currently she is working on her undergraduate honors thesis: Biophilic Design and the Mental Wellness of University Students. In this project, Susie is working with the Hayden Library Renovations Project at ASU to apply principles of biophilic design to their new mental wellness/meditation room. The goal is to create a room whose design allows for relaxation and enhances opportunity for mental dexterity and focus of students. She is also working with The Ecstasis Club at ASU on developing research focused on altered states of consciousness. Outside of academia, Susie has a love for reading, creative writing, dancing, and developing her capacity to love herself and others.

Printed by Printforce, the Netherlands